AF419196

Herbs For Children~
An easy to use parent's guide to blending safe herbal remedies

Michele Wildflower
HHP, CCC, RM

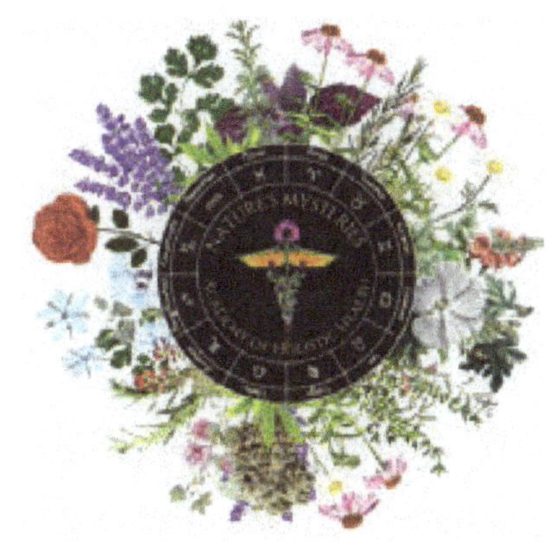

Dedication

I would like to dedicate this book to my daughters, my husband and all those who are seeking the truth. To those who don't know where to turn, who want to live a healthy life or who want to help a loved one feel better and to parents who want to educate themselves to protect their children. With the knowledge of the material contained in this book, any discomfort or symptom should be alleviated. It is my gift to you so that you will know how to live your healthiest, most vibrant life enjoying the gifts you've been given with the knowledge of how to prepare the remedies from Mother Nature's Pantry if the time comes. If your loved one, being human or pet has cancer, don't give up! I compiled much of this for you. Knowledge Is Power.

"Never doubt that a small group of thoughtful, committed citizens can change the world; indeed, it's the only thing that ever has."

— Margaret Mead

Copyright © 2020 by M. Wildflower
All Rights reserved.

No part of this book may be reproduced in any form or by any electronic or mechanical means, including information storage and retrieval systems, without written permission from the author, except for the use of brief quotations in a book review.

Acknowledgments

First, I'd like to thank my husband, Iggy Wildflower, my best friend, who ignited the spark for my quest of seeking out natural alternatives to raise our girls by gifting me a homeopathy correspondence course for my 30th birthday. And for always standing by my side, learning with me, processing everything that comes into my reality and guiding me to make sense of it all, I couldn't have done this without your never-ending, unconditional love and support.

I'd like to thank my four daughters: Marijah, Cherisse, Amareena and Isabel for giving me a reason to seek better alternatives. For showing me not only the amazing joy and love that only you could bring but for all that you've taught me and continue to teach me every day, I am so grateful.

I want to thank Dr. Paul Fanny of The University of Natural Health for asking me to write an Herbal Course, hence my book and the freedom to pass on my knowledge to the world in my own way.

And lastly, my patients and customers who trust me with their health, it is an honor to serve you and I appreciate all that you've taught me, this journey would not have been possible without your lessons and affirmations that I am on the right track.

Thank you, Everyone!

About the Author

Michele Wildflower, Holistic Health Practitioner, Director of Education at Nature's Mysteries Academy of Holistic Health, Founder and Formulator for Nature's Mysteries Apothecary, has been utilizing plant medicine for healing for over 30 years.

As a Homeopath, Herbalist, Reiki Master, Essential Oil Coach, Clinical Cannabinoid Clinician, Graduate of The Clinical Cannabinoid Medicine Curriculum, Nutritionist, Certified in Complementary and Alternative Medicine, working towards a Ph.D. in Holistic Natural Health and Nutrition, Michele is passionate about plant medicine and loves to pass on the knowledge.

Other books Michele has written:
Discover The Essence Of Cannabis Medicine ~
The Lifesaving Principles

Discover The Essence Of Plant Medicine,
The Five Principles Of Lifesaving Herbs

The Mysteries Of Medicinal Mushrooms,
Discover The Lifesaving Secrets

Understanding the importance of incorporating specific plant compounds for certain symptom management to obtain overall health, Michele details the uses and properties of 7 different herbs she has used on her healing journey, mentioning a few others along the way.

Medicinal Disclaimer

It is the policy of mine not to advise or recommend herbs for medicinal or health use. This information is intended for educational purposes only and should not be considered as a recommendation or an endorsement of any particular medical or health treatment.

Table of Contents

Introduction

Some herb books begin with stories of how the Herbalist spent time as a child in the woods or on a farm or with a loved one who shared their knowledge of plants with them. My story is not your typical Herbalist's story. I grew up in Chicago, surrounded by cement buildings, few trees, and a strip of grass separated by sidewalk and street.

No one I knew ever taught me anything about the uses of plants growing up. As a child, I would always look at nature calendars and long to sit by the brook in the picture or in that field of flowers. My longing for Nature was real. My favorite place to go was the forest preserve. It was about 20 minutes from our house, a little piece of woods that was left with trails through it that we would visit sometimes, on the weekends, for a picnic or to let the dogs run.

I remember in my early 20's meeting someone who explained that they didn't feed their children white sugar. What? Why? I had never heard of such a thing. What was wrong with sugar? So bad that a child could NEVER have it?

Over the next few years, I learned about home births, another concept I had never heard of and thought only existed in the old days. *You can have babies at home'* was my astonished response. Learning new concepts and stepping 'out of the box' became a passion.

To explore the other side, I was anxious to integrate this new outlook, this new knowledge, these new 'natural living' concepts into my own life. I started learning about diet, plants, Herbal Healing, the bounty that Mother Earth has to share with us.

I moved to Vermont when I was 23 and met my husband, at 26, I gave birth to my first daughter at home after laboring for 36 hours, choosing herbs and aqua therapy (baths) over orthodox medicine, I just waited it out. At this point, I was not the Holistic Health Practitioner that I am today, but I did know one thing. I trusted Nature and my body.

I have a woman's body. We've been giving birth for millions of years; I knew if I just trusted my body that it would know what to do. I spent a great deal of time preparing for this day, eating the right foods in the right quantities, eliminating anything that might possibly damage my fetus, taking my prenatals, practicing prenatal yoga, going for long walks, every day. A midwife once told me to look at giving birth as if I were training for an athletic event.

Over the next four years, I birthed two more baby girls at home. After my first, my midwife said, "The next one will take about 12 hours and if you have another, it will be half of that." Really? She called it! She was a very wise woman. I knew I wanted to be like her, not a midwife but an Herbalist, someone who is well versed with our plant allies and all of the gifts they have to share.

In the following years of my daughters' childhood, I researched plants and natural remedies, when my girls were sick, I would turn to Mother Nature instead of a pediatrician. With a natural remedy curing the ail, I would say, 'Well, that's another notch on the natural healing belt.' As the years progressed, I turned to Nature, every time, whether it was a Homeopathic Remedy or a tea blend I steeped, the results were the same - Radiant Health.

Over time, as I learned the many uses of plants and how to incorporate them into my life, I wanted to have a huge herb garden. Herbs seemed like Mother Nature's Pharmacy. Like, really, there's a toothache plant? Yes, there really is! Spilanthes is known for relieving the pain associated with a toothache as is Clove.

To think that plants could elicit certain reactions within my body associated with individual body parts was fascinating to me, so I started studying any herb book I could get my hands on, became part of book clubs where I received mad discounts for ordering quantities of books. And I just submerged myself into the world of herbs and discovering the essence of plant medicine. It resonated with every cell in my body. I knew this was the healing mankind needed, not pharmaceutical drugs with their plethora of side effects. Then I started researching sources.

I knew I wanted the best medicine in the purest form I could find. I found the best seed suppliers and ordered what would be my first future herb garden.

That spring came, I dug up the earth, prepared my soil for seed, planted them by the cosmic rhythms of the planets when it was optimal according to my zone and my BioDynamic planting calendar, and anxiously awaited the birth of my new garden!

As their little heads popped up out of the ground, two leaves became four and they got taller and taller. I started noticing how much they resembled the weeds I was plucking and how much they resembled the weeds that lived outside the garden.

Many of the plants I had spent hours imploring through herb books to find just the right exact ones, already grew in my backyard, literally! I had ordered Valerian, Yarrow, Burdock, St. John's wort, Plantain, Self-heal, Chamomile. As I started plucking the weeds and realizing that many of them were identical or very similar to what I planted, I started feeling like every plant has a purpose.

There is so much medicine in any one field or the forest, so much medicine in the jungle, even the ocean offering us seaweed, the Earth's bounty is medicine!

Over the next 30 years in my research, revelations and experiences with plants, I realized that there is a plant for whatever ails you. When I think of herbs I think of medicine, when I think of medicine I think of plants, when I think of plants, I don't differentiate whether they're considered a fruit, vegetable, herb, bark, resin, etc.

To me, if it's a healing plant it's an herb, however you classify it. And whether it's classified as an herb, vegetable, flower, etc., it is a living entity that we now know has emotions that can be received by equipment that confirm plants enjoy human interaction. They expel energy when attention is focused on them, physically or mentally matters not. They even feel our intention and judgments towards them. So when we tend our gardens, planting our seeds, moving our little seedlings to their home in our garden, if we look at them and treat them and even think of them as such, our success in the garden will be rewarded with an abundance of flourishing, prolific plants which is the goal if we are planning on using these extracts for medicine.

At first, I turned to the plants with the hope that they'd help, a few years in, I was continuously impressed over and over with the results. While parents around me were giving their children baby aspirin, Benadryl and Tylenol, I was giving mine Echinacea and Homeopathic Remedies.

I watched as their children needed antibiotics and multiple trips to the doctor and mine enjoyed quick recoveries. I remember one time at my Homeopath's office when my girls had a cough and cold and I asked him, in earnest, why they got sick, "I don't feed them any white sugar, they eat all organic…" His answer was, "Michele, kids get sick. Look at them."

When we looked at them, they were laughing and teasing each other, pushing each other off of the chairs, joking around, being silly. He said, "If that's what they look like when they're sick, you have nothing to worry about. It's when they are bedridden or end up in the hospital that you need to start worrying." My girls never took any prescription or over-the-counter medication, ever…their whole childhood. With plenty of illnesses experienced and they were never hospitalized, so, I know it can be done.

Clearly, if there's a broken bone, conventional medicine has a time and a place, as with any kind of trauma. But with most childhood maladies, it really doesn't. None of those 'children's' medications have ever been tested on children, it would be unethical and illegal.

So, we give them to our children, anyway, trusting our doctors' advice like so many do. But do you know there are actually 1000's of people that die every year from properly prescribed medications? Literally, way over 100,000! It varies from year to year, generally in the hundreds of thousands. Yes, from properly prescribed medications! That means they did not OD on them, they took them as instructed by their doctor.

I don't want to spend too much time on this I just want to give you something to think about. Included is a section on herbal remedies for children. Because children are so sensitive, Homeopathic doses are effective even at their minuscule levels of active compounds.

As my daughters grew, witnessing my passion for the plant kingdom and natural healing unfold, for my 30 yr old birthday, my husband gave me a Distance Learning homeopathy Course allowing me to acquire my certificate in Homeopathy and further my knowledge of plants.

Over the next few years, I also became an Herbalist, certified in Complementary and Alternative Medicine, a Reiki Master, an Essential Oil Coach, a Clinical Cannabinoid Clinician, took a Clinical Kinesiology class, I also became a candidate for a Ph.D. in Holistic Natural Health and Nutrition with The University of Natural Health, each one fueling my yearning for Holistic Healing.

My daughters grew into beautiful, healthy, young women, with no allergies or other health issues. Everyone enjoyed extreme health until 2016, when we were blindsided. My husband was diagnosed with a Triple Hit of Non-Hodgkin's Lymphoma.

Giving him only a 35% chance of curing it with their methods, predicting imminent death and advice to get his affairs in order, prompted me to relentlessly, tirelessly research cancer, the kind he had, various modalities for healing, various cancer treatments, survivor stories, prevention, etc.

My research directed me towards specific remedies, I gathered about 20 different vitamins, herbs, enzymes, minerals, mushrooms and we had it gone in about three months, to his Oncologist's dismay! She allowed him to take the supplementation I provided alongside her five day long, IV, inpatient chemo treatments.

They complemented each other, if you will. The herbs guiding the chemo to where it needed to go. This is what my logo is for Nature's Mysteries Apothecary, all of the plants that my husband used to rid his body of cancer. Every time we go back for a check-up, she will reiterate that he's cured and that the kind of cancer he had definitely would have come back by now!

Incorporating more than just the plant kingdom, but the mineral kingdom as well as pancreatic enzymes, Mindfulness Techniques, proper diet, eliminating certain foods and drinks as well as toxic people and environments was a lot of work, but very worth it in the end!

There are so many cures for cancer now and so many more being found every day that are natural that do not wage war on our bodies. As a cancer patient, love and nourishment are what is required, not being subjected to a rendezvous with death, coming as close as possible and feeling what the repercussions of that feel like. Our bodies prefer plant compounds over chemicals; they know how to synthesize these organic molecules.

In this book, we will learn about herbs and natural therapies and their origins, such as Bach Flower Remedies and Homeopathy, a basic history of herbs is included to give the reader background and basis for understanding the world of Holistic Herbal Healing, methods of preparation, and uses for each plant.

Information is provided on how to prescribe and treat symptoms with herbs, the difference between prescribing and diagnosing. We will delve into the differences between native plants and cultivars, chemical, synthetic, single molecule medicine and plant medicine. Learn why medicine from Nature has a whole host of benefits instead of a long list of side effects.

You will have a basic understanding of how and when it shifted from natural herbal medicine to chemical medications. We will learn about The Law of Opposites, Doctrine of Signatures, Traditional Chinese Medicine, Ayurvedic Medicine, the Simpler's Method, Cancer Prevention and Alternative Treatments, Mindfulness Techniques, a whole section devoted to the Hemp/Cannabis plant, what Cannabinoids are, the role of our Endocannabinoid System, the vital connection between mind and body, new groundbreaking brain research, the mysteries of mushrooms and safe alternatives for children.

The plant kingdom is so vast, depending on the area you live and your native plants that I couldn't possibly mention in detail every plant that I love in this book or it would be too heavy to carry around. So, what I will do is mention plants that I know of that will help specific ailments, but we will go into detail for 7 that I have utilized over the years and have had great success with and I'm sure you will too!

"Medicine is not only a science; it is also an art. It does not consist of compounding pills and plasters; it deals with the very processes of life, which must be understood before they may be guided." — *Paracelsus*

Herbs for Children

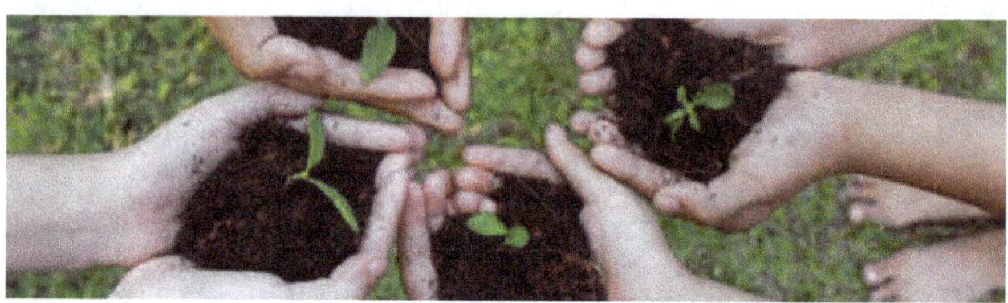

"Kids know this intuitively. It's simply the culture we've been mostly raised in here in this part of the world that either ignored it, or actively repressed it. But probably the dire straits we're in now are awakening more people to it, frankly. That this is real, and is not some airy-fairy thing. It's real that plants have energy and personality and they have gifts, and we need to honor them, and we're here all together on the same level. No one's more important than anybody else. We work in synergy."

— Annie McCleary

In this book, we will learn the value of choosing plants over poison for our family. Never having been tested on children, we offer over-the-counter and pharmaceutical medications to our babies, who are trusting us, trusting our doctor's advice. But what if what the pediatrician is recommending, doesn't feel right?

Understanding how your child's whole future lies on the decisions we make today and grasping the importance of reading thoroughly anything before we give it to our children will be understood.

We'll explore the toxic toys that are made for us to give to our children knowing that they will put them in their mouth, as well as the BPA-laden plastic baby bottles, nipples, sippy cups, etc. An even deeper knowledge will be transferred as to the life-threatening effects of formula.

A basic understanding of viruses and how they invade your child's body will be put forth, with natural antibiotic options that you might not have thought of, especially thinking of them as being antibiotic. The concepts surrounding sickness and possible reasons your child gets sick will be explored as well as possible immune boosters that you can provide them to build their immune system without damaging their gut flora and causing a plethora of side effects while breaking down their immune system.

We'll delve into treatments for rashes, coughs, fevers, nightmares, etc. with practical methods for treating these maladies and recipes included. Understanding that we are energetic beings and the possible dangers and an awareness of the detrimental health effects a cell phone can cause to the developing brain of a child will be given.

The concept of sugary sweets and how they can ruin your child's taste buds with constructive ways to get your children to eat properly are suggested. Along with recipes for healthy treats that your children will not only love and enjoy making but will wish they could have more of, which will be fine with you because they are good for them!

We will be introduced to Dr. Maria Montessori and grasp what she has done for children and the state of childhood all over the world. A guide to the most important plant allies to have in your First Aid Kit as well as ideas on how to make recovery time a breeze after injuries and trauma are included.

Chapter 1 ~ What You Need to Know

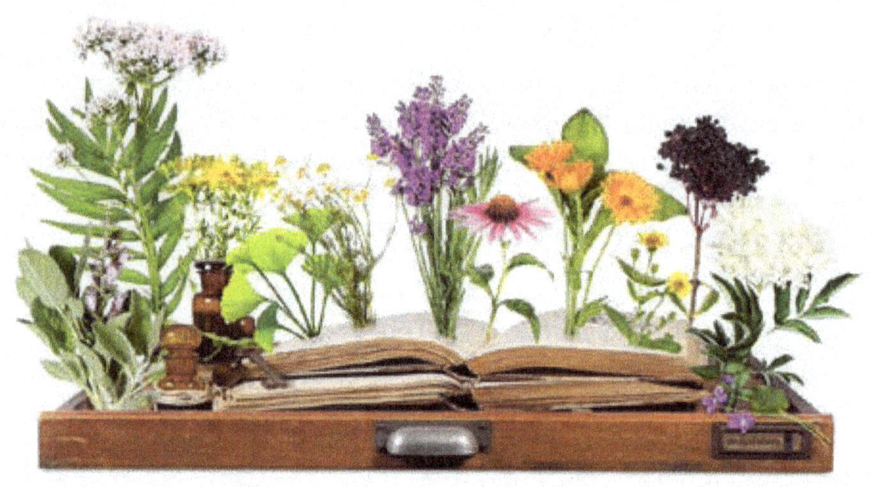

"Encourage your child to have muddy, grassy or sandy feet by the end of each day, that's the childhood they deserve."

- Penny Whitehouse

New Chapter Prenatals

All prenatals are not created equally and are far from being the same, don't listen to anybody who tells you differently. If this is your first pregnancy, now's the perfect time to start understanding that you need to think for yourself, listen to no one, and read the heck out of labels, at every turn!

A prenatal that your conventional doctor from the hospital will prescribe for you will not be plant-based, will not be easily absorbed, will have several 'possible side effects' that are more like 'direct effects.' So, what can you do?

New Chapter is a company I trust that prepares its vitamins from fermented food. So not only are they made from organic whole foods, but they have been fermented to ensure proper absorption and assimilation. And they also include nourishing herbs that will tone and establish vital compounds preparing your body for the amazing act of giving birth.

This is just my suggestion, ensuring that they are organic, fermented and made with whole food would be some of the criteria that I would be looking for in a vitamin. (I would also recommend finding a local midwife if you don't already have one to complement your birthing process.) Midwife appointments are very different from a doctor's appointment and I think you will find them quite enjoyable.

Two Choices

Waking up in the middle of the night to your little loved one crying from discomfort from a fever, or unable to breathe or to stop coughing, or worse, vomiting, is one of the worst ways to wake up, the only thought in your mind is comforting them and giving them something to calm them down and bring relief.

We have two choices: To either administer children's Tylenol, which has never been tested on children, much less babies, (that would be unethical) to stop the fever or the cough, while possibly damaging our child's liver and kidneys, taxing their immune system and most importantly stopping their bodies' natural defense mechanism to fight pathogens when it's under attack.

Also containing sucralose which destroys their gut bacteria that they will likely need to fight off whatever pathogen has invaded their system and let's not forget the artificial colors which are known to cause behavioral issues in children, among other things. Then we could set them up in front of the TV or a video game with a soda and some artificially colored orange chips and call it good.

Or you could brew some tea for them, give them a spoonful of honey (for children over 1 year of age), rub some mentholated salve you made on their chest, reach for the Elderberry cough syrup you made or bought and give them a gentle Homeopathic Remedy suited for their discomfort that will not hinder their natural defenses, but enhance them. Read them a book, cuddle up on the couch, maybe put on some soft music, turn on the salt lamp, increasing the negative ions in the room.

The choice is yours. Either way, you are going to have to get up, so it's not really like one is any easier than the other. But one will play a significant role in the health and well-being, vitality and longevity that your child enjoys throughout their life.

But No Pressure

Being a parent is a heavy responsibility; our decisions are the deciding factors of this child's immunity for their whole life. But no pressure. We, as their parents are going to be the result of them having allergies that bother them for their whole life, asthma, digestive issues, etc.

It's all in our hands. It is our obligation as a parent to educate ourselves BEFORE we administer ANYTHING to our children, to not follow suit because our neighbor said she gives it to her child all of the time and said nothing's ever happened.

Another Notch on the Natural Healing Belt!

I remember one time when my middle daughter, Amareena, was little (22 years ago) and she had a rash that we could not get rid of. She had little bumps that started on her legs and just increased. I was not the Herbalist I am today and when my trusty Weleda Diaper Rash Creme didn't work and they kept coming out, we went to the doctor.

At this time, we didn't have any doctor, natural or otherwise, because we enjoyed health, so we went to the closest place just to see what it was. They didn't know and referred us to a Dermatologist at Dartmouth to try to get to the bottom of it.

They were not much help at all, but they did give us a creme that she told me to '...rub all over her body but just make sure that you don't get it on her face,' were the instructions. "What, why not," I asked? "Because it could hurt...the skin on the face is sensitive so it's better kept off of the face." She almost said it could hurt her face!

I don't know if she didn't notice that my daughter's face was attached to her body, I'm thinking if it could hurt her face, why wouldn't it hurt the rest of her body? We took it home never intending to use it. The rash kept getting worse and my husband said to me, "What are you going to do about it? If it was on her face, you wouldn't let it go this long…"

I didn't know what to do, I really didn't, never having dealt with this before. So, we rubbed that ointment on her, and as I rubbed it on, feeling horrible the whole time, he started reading the side effects. I had rubbed a little on her knee and he said, "It says something about causing cranium damage or something like that!"

"What?" I grabbed it from his hand and he said, "Why did you put it on her?" I was like, "You just told me to!" So, you get where I'm going with this, always make sure that you read the label first if you choose to use any kind of pharmaceutical medication.

We chose not to risk her cranium or whatever it was and I started researching. It was a nice April that year, with lots of sunshine, living remotely and having a big yard, I let her run around naked outside in the Sun, she was 2 so she loved every minute of it.

For a couple of hours a day, getting that fresh air and Sun, living in Vermont, come April, her skin hadn't seen any Sun in a long time. I started giving her long colloidal oatmeal baths every day and rubbing a natural lotion on her that did not contain any synthetic ingredients after the bath. Within 2 weeks, the rash was gone! Another notch on the 'Natural Healing Belt!'

Amareena's Rash That Wouldn't Go Away Recipe

- 2 hours Sunlight every day with no sunscreen with as much skin exposed as possible

- Colloidal oatmeal baths every day - long soaks, follow directions on package

- Organic lotion or herbal oils applied two times a day, one after bath

- Repeat this for two weeks or until you see signs of improvement

Read Labels

We need to read labels, this human being's life and longevity are in our hands. Lack of information and ignorance can result in a myriad of disorders and diseases that could have been avoided through knowledge. Education of what we're eating, what we're wearing, what process takes place when manufacturing these products. What kind of residue is left behind? What are the possible implications of our actions? We need answers to these questions.

Toxic Baby Toys

So many baby and toddler toys are actually made with plastics that are completely carcinogenic. Like those little rubber duckies? Yes, you know the ones, completely toxic! Those soft squishy toys utilize a specific kind of plastic to make them soft, called PVC. The majority of plastics used to make children's toys contain carcinogens (cancer-causing compounds.)

Here is a list of toxic ingredients found in PVC according to Green Child Magazine.

Harmful Additives to PVC

- **Phthalates** (pronounced thay-lates) give a plastic toy its soft, squishy feel. These are the gender-bending culprits you've heard of, endocrine disruptors. Phthalates not only upset the body's hormonal balance, they've also been found to stimulate the growth of cancers.

- **Cadmium** is a plastic stabilizer. A known carcinogen, cadmium also affects normal brain growth and can cause kidney damage.

- **Lead** is used to make plastic toys more durable. Lead affects the nervous system and has been linked to hearing loss, ADHD and decreased IQ. It's also a concern because children absorb and retain lead in their systems more easily than adults.

BPA (Bisphenol A) is found in plastic toys, sippy cups, plastic bottles and canned food lining. It's considered more of a danger when the child chews on it, so the main concern with BPA has been on food and drink products. But if your child is prone to chewing on toys (and what baby isn't?) it's best to avoid plastic toys for that stage.

Here's the link to that article:

https://www.greenchildmagazine.com/plastic-toys/

Lead

The paint used to paint these toys (even on the wooden toys) often has lead in it. The toys in the gumball machines are made with lead. Not even kidding! Read this article from CBS News about a little 4-year-old boy who swallowed a trinket from a gumball machine and absorbed 12 times the normal level of lead in his bloodstream, enough to nearly killing him! You can read about it here:

https://www.cbsnews.com/news/gumball-trinkets-dangerous-charms/

While there have been recalls it's really not that much better, this just gives you an idea of the kind of underhandedness that is afoot degrading the quality of your child's toys!!! This should be enough to get you started researching this…when our girls were little, we only bought cloth, natural rubber or wooden toys, but then I learned that the paint on them is made with lead. Do you see how they do that? It's no mistake, even if you try to be conscious, they are trying to undermine your best efforts. Why??

That's why I started turning to the UK, paints coming out of Germany on children's toys are nontoxic. Thailand has a few good companies, too, that I have included as well as other reputable companies that actually care about your child's health and longevity. They are a little more expensive, but I guess that's the price we pay for non-endocrine disrupting toys.

Believe me, I really wish it wasn't this way, but maybe if we all stop buying these toxic toys, they'll stop selling them. Our dollar is our most powerful voice, let's direct our voice where we want it to be heard and where it will have the loudest most resounding effect...in the shareholders' pockets... you have to 'hit them where it hurts'... to get their attention.

Paraffin Wax

Ready for this? Kid's sidewalk chalk has lead in it. You are definitely going to want to make sure that if you buy this for your children that it is lead-free. Crayons have been found to have lead in them, too! But that's not even all of it, many commercial crayon companies (e.g., Crayola) are making crayons mainly from paraffin wax, which is a derivative of petroleum.

Starting out as a grayish-black sludge left over after the petroleum refining process, after all of the other petroleum-based products (gas, pavement, oil) have been removed. Then being bleached and processed, both of these steps require the use of toxic chemicals.

Generally considered to be non-toxic but the process of producing paraffin certainly isn't! But that still isn't even the worst of it, as if lead and paraffin aren't enough, let's just throw in some asbestos, too?

Come on, all of this in our children's toys?? So sad...so so sad...so true.

Asbestos

Here's an article from CBS News:

'Parents buying school supplies for grammar schoolers would be wise to avoid Playskool crayons. The brand, sold at Dollar Tree, was found to have trace elements of asbestos.'

"The good news is that when we were testing three years ago, all sorts of brands came back with asbestos," said Kara Cook-Schultz, toxics director at U.S. Public Interest Research Group, which conducts annual tests of toys and school supplies. "Now it's just this one."

'Indeed, in tests run in 2015, many major brands, including Disney Mickey Mouse Clubhouse Crayons and Nickelodeon Teenage Mutant Ninja Turtles crayons, contained trace amounts of asbestos fibers — a substance that can cause breathing difficulties and cancer if inhaled.'

'*Although the Consumer Product Safety Commission acknowledged that it was unclear whether the asbestos trapped in crayon wax posed a danger,* it noted that kids sometimes eat crayons and recommended that parents avoid asbestos-containing brands as a precaution.'

Can we just read that part again… 'the Consumer Product Safety Commission acknowledged that it was UNCLEAR whether the ASBESTOS trapped IN CRAYON wax posed a DANGER,' are you serious right now? They are 'unclear' whether asbestos really poses a danger to your child when it's in their hand? These are the people protecting us? Need I say more about this? I think I'm just going to leave that one right there.

Here's a list of companies you can trust -

Non-toxic Alternative Art Supplies:

- **Beeswax**
- **Lepze Crayons**
- **Crayon Rocks**
- **Gibot Toddler**
- **Aquarelle**
- **Lyra**
- **Faber Castell**
- **Stockmar**

Some of My Favorite Non-toxic Toy Companies:

- **HABA**
- **Oompa**
- **Plan Toys**
- **Camden Rose**
- **Grimm's Spiel and Holz**
- **Spielstabil**
- **Under The Nile**

- **Wonderworld**

Silicone Nipples/Glass Baby Bottles

Not to mention the nipples on bottles for babies who are not breastfed, that are drinking out of toxic plastic bottles, whose mothers are heating up their formula in microwaves. NEVER HEAT A BABY BOTTLE IN A MICROWAVE!!

So not only is the microwaved liquid changing the baby's blood (refer to the section about Microwave Radiation), but when heated, plastic leaches toxins found in the plastics into their drink.

This is why they say don't drink out of water bottles that have sat in the sun that contain BPA because the heat from the sun causes it to leach into the water. Or how about the plastics that pacifiers are made with, sippy cups, etc.?

We used glass bottles for my grandson when I babysat him, not wanting to trust plastics. For nipples, we went with silicone. And that's what I'd recommend, either that or natural rubber if you can find it.

Potential Harm

It's not our fault that everything being offered to us could potentially damage our child's endocrine system, that the majority of formulas out there don't even contain any food. If you read the label, there's not a lot of plant ingredients in there, with GMO sugars and so many corn and soy type of ingredients.

And if there's dairy, it's dairy that you know is from cows treated with rbST or rbGH/Bovine growth hormone (recombinant bovine somatotropin) given to cows to increase their milk production. As stated in the second chapter.

Approved in 1993 by the FDA. Cows treated with this hormone began developing so many significant health issues including a 50% increase in the risk of lameness (leg and hoof problems), over a 25% increase in the frequency of udder infections (mastitis), and serious animal reproductive problems, such as infertility, cystic ovaries, fetal loss and birth defects. But do you think the FDA pulled it? Or even made mandatory labeling?

No. I remember when this happened in Vermont. We pushed so hard for labeling that I remember walking down the aisle in the store and any dairy product containing this growth hormone had a little blue dot by its price tag. The ENTIRE dairy aisle had one on it. Except for Cabot and Butterworks, they were the only companies that didn't have that blue dot. Well, let me tell you, that didn't last long! That went away and then it took years to get the labeling on each product.

Formula Risks

Here is a list of ingredients from one of the leading formula companies who shall remain nameless: should I say it's Enfamil?

NONFAT MILK, LACTOSE, VEGETABLE OIL (PALM OLEIN, COCONUT, SOY, AND HIGH OLEIC SUNFLOWER OILS), WHEY PROTEIN CONCENTRATE, AND LESS THAN 2%:

GALACTOOLIGOSACCHARIDES*, POLYDEXTROSE*,

MORTIERELLA ALPINA OIL†, CRYPTHECODINIUM COHNII

OIL‡, CALCIUM CARBONATE, POTASSIUM CITRATE, FERROUS SULFATE, POTASSIUM CHLORIDE, MAGNESIUM OXIDE, SODIUM CHLORIDE, ZINC SULFATE, CUPRIC SULFATE,

MANGANESE SULFATE, POTASSIUM IODIDE, SODIUM

SELENITE, SOY LECITHIN, CHOLINE CHLORIDE, ASCORBIC

ACID, NIACINAMIDE, CALCIUM PANTOTHENATE, VITAMIN A

PALMITATE, VITAMIN B12, VITAMIN D3, RIBOFLAVIN, THIA-MIN HYDROCHLORIDE, VITAMIN B6 HYDROCHLORIDE,

FOLIC ACID, VITAMIN K1, BIOTIN, INOSITOL, VITAMIN E

ACETATE, NUCLEOTIDES (CYTIDINE 5'-MONOPHOSPHATE,

DISODIUM URIDINE 5'-MONOPHOSPHATE, ADENOSINE 5'MONOPHOSPHATE, DISODIUM GUANOSINE 5'MONO-PHOSPHATE), TAURINE, L-CARNITINE.

Reviews

If you go read the 8 reviews just on the first page, 5 out of the 8 say that their baby either had such severe reactions to the powder, that they tried the liquid or that it upset their child's stomach, that it gave them gas, bloating, constipation, discomfort, diarrhea...go look, I couldn't make this stuff up.

You know that all of those vitamins are synthetic, the dairy is tainted with growth hormones, antibiotics, rendered feed, not to mention rich in glutamines (which we learned about in the Glutamate section) and GMO corn and soy, (which we learned about in the GMO section.)

Poor babies don't have a chance if they are not breast-fed and even if they are and their mothers are toxic then it is passed down to them through the milk, such as with nicotine or alcohol. When my girls were babies and they were sick, since you can't administer teas or tinctures to babies, I would ingest it knowing that my daughter would reap the benefit of it being passed through my milk.

I would like to 'throw' some facts at you, if you will, so you can make your own educated decision without even having to put down this book to do some research. I have included some very thorough research done from all over the world and what the findings reveal is that your baby is better off without formula. Instead of giving you the research and then the conclusions, I've started with the conclusions and then you can see how they based these conclusions. It is definitely something worth looking into, I'd say, to say the least, especially if you are considering feeding your baby formula…

This information is gathered from Dr. Linda Palmer, an advocate for natural parenting techniques. Her extensive reviews of science and medical research revealed huge conflicts between what is found scientifically and what is standard protocol in pediatric offices.

Her research in this area led to writing *Baby Matters*. After an IPPY award-winning 2nd edition, the 3rd updated edition was released by Sourcebooks as *The Baby Bond*. After a print-run sell-out, *Baby Matters* has returned, as the 3rd revised edition (same as The Baby Bond).

Palmer also co-authored another infant health book with pediatrician Susan Markel: *What Your Pediatrician Doesn't Know Can Hurt Your Child*.

Formula Research Conclusion
What your doctor doesn't tell you.

Pediatricians spend much time frightening parents with 1 in 100,000 risks from some vaccine-preventable diseases when parents question the utility and safety of vaccines. 'Would you want to risk the life of your child?' they demand. Yet these very same professionals offer formula samples with the other hand — when the magnitude of health risks associated with the use of formula is five times greater.

Parenting is all about making choices and weighing risks and benefits. Many parents need to make the riskier choice of formula feeding in order to balance other factors that benefit the family. Yet some parents who have lost their children, possibly based on pediatric advice condoning or encouraging formula-feeding, would surely wish that they had been informed of the very real risks related to using formula.

So now we are left to examine artificial feeding's actual impact on all American babies. First, we note that there should be a relationship dictating that if rates for a certain disease are doubled by formula feeding, for instance, then death rates for that disease may also be somewhere in the neighborhood of doubled when compared with rates for breastfed infants. In fact, the evidence suggests that the death rates would be even higher.

While formula feeding may result in twice as many episodes of a certain illness, a great number of studies demonstrate that each of these episodes are also longer and more severe. This would suggest that the rate of death among artificially fed infants from various causes would actually be higher than the rates that the various illnesses occur. Twenty-two nations with high rates of breastfeeding have infant mortality rates below 5, while the U.S. ranks higher in infant death than 41 other nations. Clearly, lower rates for the United States are a possibility.

It's commonly said that formula feeding does not risk lives in industrialized nations where education and medical advances prevent increased deaths. The evidence is quite to the contrary. Some insist that the blame for the United States' relatively high infant death rate lies with underprivileged communities. Again, it has been shown that elevated death rates among U.S. blacks cannot be attributed to poverty. Hispanic Americans rank similarly to African-American populations for socioeconomic factors, but they match non-Hispanic whites in their lower infant mortality rates. The difference is not socioeconomic; rather, it's in rates of formula use versus breastfeeding.

A New York study sought to establish the connection between education, income and infant survival. It concluded strongly that the number of illnesses is increased by two to three times in formula-fed babies regardless of socioeconomic status or level of parental education. A later study in Israel confirmed the effects of formula feeding across all classes and education levels. The most recent analysis of this issue, again performed in the United States, reiterated that higher illness rates among formula-fed or formula-supplemented infants 'did not differ among income groups.' In fact, an increased risk of death throughout life has been well documented for people who were formula-fed. Higher blood pressure, more heart disease, obesity, diabetes and artery disease, a nearly doubled rate of Crohn's disease and tripled rates of celiac disease have all been associated with early formula feeding.

Translate actually to 56% more infant deaths for those receiving mostly formula. A relative risk of 13 here means that a child who was not breastfed through the time period has thirteen times the risk of dying during his first year as a child who had received any breast milk through that period. A relative risk of 5 here means that an infant who receives formula statistically faces five times the risk of dying as an infant who is partially or completely breastfed.

Sudden Infant Death Syndrome (SIDS)

Sudden Infant Death Syndrome (SIDS) accounts for a full 10% of U.S. infant deaths. Several studies performed in the United States and other industrialized nations reveal increased risks of SIDS among babies who receive formula instead of breast milk. In the table below, the 2002 Scandinavian study takes into account variables thought to have affected the 2000 U.S. study, finding even stronger risks associated with formula.

The most recent U.S. study (2003) takes advantage of the lessons from these earlier studies to raise confidence in its final results. Its finding of five times the risk of infant death from SIDS for formula-fed infants seems to be the most powerful statistic yet. A relative risk of 5 here means that an infant who receives formula statistically faces five times the risk of dying from SIDS as an infant who is breastfed.

Heart, Circulatory and Respiratory Failure

Premature infants and those with circulatory abnormalities often display one or more warning signs of potential death, including inadequate oxygenation of the blood, apnea (episodes where breathing stops) and high blood pressure. Studies illustrate the dangers of formula for these infants. One study observed better body temperature and superior oxygenation in pre-term infants receiving breast milk. Formula-fed infants demonstrated many episodes of inadequate oxygenation and some apnea, both of which were not seen among the breastfed infants. A Scottish study found significantly better blood pressure among naturally fed infants.

Three U.S. studies are available examining feeding methods for infants with early circulatory problems. One study reported that more than half of infants with congenital heart disease lost oxygenation during bottle feedings, while none did so while breastfeeding. Another study also dealing with heart disease found infants' growth to be significantly inferior and their hospitalizations to be longer when they were fed formula. A third study of very low birth-weight infants found twice as many episodes of inadequate oxygenation among formula-fed infants as in those who received breast milk.

Necrotizing Enterocolitis

Necrotizing enterocolitis is a severe intestinal inflammatory disorder that affects around 4% of low birth-weight babies and 1% of full-term infants. About one-third of low birth-weight infants and 20% of full-term infants who contract this disorder die.

While necrotizing enterocolitis is reported to be responsible for 1.4% of infant deaths, many more unconfirmed cases are likely to be responsible for some portion of infant deaths reported as caused by prematurity. In the United Kingdom, it was discovered that confirmed cases of necrotizing enterocolitis occurred in three times as many infants who received no breast milk as in those who received both breast milk and formula. For infants who exclusively received breast milk, necrotizing enterocolitis occurred six to 10 times less often than among wholly formula-fed infants.

Diarrhea

A World Health Organization (WHO) study revealed a risk of diarrhea for formula-fed babies in developing nations averaging more than six times that of breastfed babies. A summary article for industrialized nations demonstrated an average of triple the risk of diarrhea for formula-fed babies. The risk in China and Israel is reported as slightly less than triple (2.8); in Scotland, the risk is five-fold; and a doubled risk is measured in Canada.

While one study noted nearly twice the risk of developing diarrhea for artificially fed infants in Brazil, other studies have demonstrated that the risk of actually dying from diarrhea was an astounding 14 to 15 times greater. The latter studies demonstrated not only that the artificially fed infants suffer higher rates of illness, but also that the severity and duration of their illnesses are even greater when they do occur and result in proportionately more deaths. This same assertion is demonstrated in a study from India, where formula-fed infants suffer six times the death rate, once diarrhea occurs, as breastfed infants with diarrhea.

Four separate studies in the United States all deduce a doubled risk of diarrhea for formula-fed babies. The U.S. studies also reiterate the well established factor of greater severity and extent of illness once diarrhea does occur among formula-fed babies. Death rates for formula-fed U.S. infants who get diarrhea may be three times higher or more than their breastfed contemporaries.

Respiratory Illnesses

Numerous studies document higher numbers of respiratory infections among formula-fed infants than among those who are breastfed. It is clear that respiratory infections are at least triple in the United States for formula-fed infants.

Congenital Abnormalities

Twenty percent of U.S. infant deaths are attributed to birth defects. The most common potentially lethal birth defects include heart disorders, various chromosomal or genetic defects and underdeveloped lungs. In terms of infant formula's impact, we have the least amount of statistical information in this category. However, many factors suggest that formula fed infants with congenital abnormalities have smaller chances of survival than their breastfed counterparts.

While death certificates often list the initial abnormality as the cause of death, infection is actually the final factor in many of these deaths. We have already seen how drastically infection rates and deaths are reduced by breastfeeding. It is clear that the youngest and weakest infants are the ones who are most strongly endangered by infant formula's inadequacies.

Studies suggest that formula-fed infants suffer inferior blood oxygenation and higher blood pressure as well as more episodes of apnea (cessation of breathing for a short time) than their breastfed counterparts. While no studies compare the actual survival of such infants in the United States, it is obvious that some proportion of babies with congenital heart abnormalities is being seriously disadvantaged by formula feedings. Artificially fed infants with heart defects requiring surgery are less likely to live until their surgery and less likely to recover from surgery's challenges.

A wide variety of common birth defects has been shown to have better survival rates among breastfed infants, although the actual figures are not available. Most birth defects have not been specifically studied in this regard. The background information, nonetheless, is striking.

For example, infants born with phenylketonuria (PKU), a defect in handling a certain protein in the diet, need specialized supplementation to breast milk in order to prevent mental retardation and other difficulties. Yet a study demonstrated that infants who had been breastfed before being diagnosed with PKU fared far better than those who had been fed on formula. The greatest complications for infants with cystic fibrosis are lung infection, decreased oxygenation and malnutrition — all of which are recognized to be complicated by formula feeding. The negative impact of formula on neurological development has been demonstrated in healthy infants. One study that quantified the effect reported double the amount of neurological 'nonnormality' in formula-fed infants. It is reasonable to assume that neurological damage or problems stemming from birth disorders can be exacerbated by artificial feeding.'

Here's the whole article:

http://babyreference.com/formula-feeding-doubles-infant-deathsin-america/

Great resource:

The Baby Bond: The New Science Behind What's Really Important When Caring for Your Baby

Premature Babies

I chose not to show the data for premature babies because I sense that if you are in the hospital with a premature baby, you are not going to have much luck giving your baby human milk. But trust me, if there was any way that it was possible, that will be your first choice over formula as soon as possible to increase your baby's chances of survival.

Feeding Baby

Earth's Best Baby Formula

This formula is an excellent alternative to conventional formulas, produced by a company who cares so that if nursing isn't an option for you or if you are trying to supplement with formula or wean your baby, this is a perfect option. Feel good knowing that you are offering the light of your eye the best that you can offer.

Almond Milk

A 2005 study conducted in Italy found that almond milk is an effective substitute of cow's milk in infants with cow milk allergy or intolerance. For the study, 52 infants with cow milk allergy or intolerance, follow this link:

https://draxe.com/nutrition/dairy-freediet/

Nursing Your Baby

So what are you supposed to do if you can't nurse, first of all, if you want to breastfeed, I wouldn't listen to anybody who tells you that you can't, I know of one woman who was told she would never be able to bear a child who had 5 babies after being told that, just to show them up.

Nobody ever met you before or has any idea what you are capable of, never let them underestimate your power, will and determination. Until I have tried every herb and herbal combination out there, I will believe there's a way.

Unless there is something literally, physically prohibiting you, herbs can be the gentle, guided support that your body needs to stimulate lactation. I knew of a woman who wanted a baby so bad who could not conceive who adopted a baby and rigged a bottle with a tube that ran along her breast so the baby would suckle to get fed and her body started producing milk from the baby suckling even though she was never pregnant!

Our bodies are AMAZING, don't ever forget the miracle you've been given. If you've tried everything to no avail, find a Midwife and seek professional help, I wouldn't give up until all avenues have been exhausted. You have a woman's body and we have been nursing our babies for eons.

If you don't want to, that is your choice, but if you want to, there are herbs that not only stimulate lactation but increase lactation. Odds are your orthodox Healthcare Provider is not aware of ANY of them and will tell you that you can't nurse.

The following herbs are called galactagogues stimulating and regulating lactation. Happy Nursing!

Choose one or a blend:

Lactation Increasing Herbs – (galactagogues)

- Marshmallow
- Nettle
- Borage
- Fenugreek
- Milk Thistle

Seeds of:

- Anise
- Caraway
- Fennel

Not Introducing Dairy Until After 2 Years Old

There is also sound evidence now, that has been around for 20 years, another one of these 'natural living concepts' that I was introduced to, that giving dairy to children under 2 years of age can actually lead to milk allergies later in life. If not as a result of an allergy to the milk protein, then an intolerance to lactose.

Not all symptoms are known or suspected as being signs of dairy allergies such as:

- **Dark circles**
- **Runny nose**
- **Sinus problems**
- **Sinus infections**
- **Postnasal drip**
- **Constant cough**
- **Clearing throat**
- **Gas**
- **Bloating**
- **Diarrhea**
- **Indigestion**
- **Ear infections**

And really, I have seen this with my own daughters, my first two were 19 months apart, close enough that one wasn't old enough to notice what the other one was doing or close enough that they could be treated similarly. These first two NEVER ate dairy the first two years, no exceptions.

The third one came 3 years later, by the time she was one, my oldest was four, plenty old enough to be enjoying ice cream especially in the summer, at the beach, living by Lake Willoughby, this happened often. So, because we were all having ice cream, my youngest would, too.

Remember, I said that my girls weren't allowed many sweets that weren't organic, but it was hormone-free, so this occasional ice cream treat when we were out was a big deal! And while nowadays, most places might even have dairy-free options, this was 20 years ago, in the North East Kingdom of Vermont, we still don't have those options up here in our town!

So naturally, we weren't about to all eat ice cream in front of Isabel, so she got a 'baby' one…and she is the only one who has dairy allergies, today.

Throughout her childhood, she'd clear her throat a lot, cough and we didn't even buy milk, we did have cheese in the house but I started buying 'raw cheese' with the enzymes intact to assist in the digestion of the cheese.

But now she is dairy-free, not eating any dairy; whereas, my other two daughters eat dairy without any problem. This is what I mean when I say our decisions will affect our child's health for the rest of their life…but no pressure.

Cow's Milk

Human babies require saturated fats as well as cholesterol in mother's milk. Bovine milk fat is nowhere near appropriately composed for human babies. The reason for this being cow's milk and its derivatives today make up one-third of the adult diet and half to two-thirds of caloric intake in children, thus replacing so much other important, nutritious food required in their diet.

This leads to insufficient intake of important healthy fiber, several minerals, vitamins and vegetable oils. Resulting in a lack of consumption of foods that are cancer-preventing, antioxidant rich foods being included in the diet. There's only so much room in there, if we fill their bellies full of milk, we are limiting the quantity available for vital nutrients that are crucial to optimum health.

Talc in Baby Powder

For the scope of this book, I am just going to tell you to trust me on this one, I don't want to spend too much time on it, but yet again, you have to be watching at every turn! Please see Annex B for information on Talc toxicity.

Best Alternatives to Talc ~

Natural Baby Powders:

- Arrowroot

- Slippery Elm

- Organic corn starch

I Choose Plants Over Poison

Allowing your child's body to fight off invaders, naturally, strengthens their immune system. Herbs can be a welcome addition to the body as fuel because the vital nutrients and compounds that are found within are crucial for the optimum functioning of the human body. Sometimes whether the body has too many toxins and is suffering from toxic overload or has had inadequate nutrition, not enough rest or sleep, too much stress, etc. can result in imbalances within your child's system.

When you choose plants over pharmaceutical medications, you are choosing to strengthen your child's body by giving them compounds that their bodies know how to synthesize, that will not cause liver or kidney damage but will actually improve the function of the liver and kidneys, as well as assisting in the processing of eliminating toxins and purifying the blood in this way enabling your child to fight properly.

Our Greatest Gift

At the end of the day, that's the goal, right? For them to have a strong immune system throughout their lives equipped to fight off any potential invaders. The greatest gift that we can give our children is a strong immune system; it's like giving them a suit of armor, protecting them even when we can't be there.

We then don't have to worry about whom they come in contact with and wonder if they are sick because we know our child is strong. We have had times when visiting family and everyone around us kept getting sick, getting on and off antibiotics, but we never got it, taking our vitamins and supplements the whole time while enjoying our sustainable organic diet. And knowing that even if we do get sick, our immune system will be stronger for it.

Shots

Every time, remember when we were kids and we got sick? No big deal, maybe you got to stay home from school, maybe you got to have some ginger ale. By the time the sickness ran its course, you were fine and back at it, bugging your parents. And that's how our immune systems build themselves.

We didn't need to inject ourselves with anything to make sure we didn't get sick. This seems to be a hysteria that has been inflicted on us by Big Pharma; that we need to inject poisons into our body to hasten getting sick.

They don't guarantee that it won't happen, so you are literally inviting poison into your child's system hoping that they will be strong enough to fight it off. But the thing is Homeopathy teaches us that for most of these shots, that we continually introduce their bodies too, that if they did even catch it, they'd be able to fight it. No problem.

If they can fight off the vaccine, then they could fight off the illness. But if they never came in contact with it, then they'd be that much the better. Instead, they want us to continuously inflict our children's immune systems with deadly diseases that were grown on animals or diseases in petri dishes, in eggs and then injected into our children introducing not only poisons, needlessly, way more than they would naturally come in contact with at one time, completely taxing their immune system, but also intermingling animal DNA with our child's DNA. Pretty sure that's not good practice. What if your child had an egg allergy?

Flu Shots

I didn't want to get into this too much, because it is such a controversial subject and I don't want to push anyone away. But while writing this course, my little 10 yr. old patient who is considered a 'fragile' child because of her condition, was given the flu shot. Not long after she came down with the flu-B virus and pneumonia putting her in the hospital and I was told that a study has begun across the country to chart this 'phenomenon' of children getting the flu after the shot. This is no 'phenomenon.' There are so many different strains of the flu going around that they can't possibly know which one will be circulating every year. So they take a guess and inject everybody with it, not hoping it works, they don't care! They got the money, that's all they care about.

Autoimmune Disease and Vaccines

It is now thought that the steady increase that we have seen in autoimmune disease has something to do with vaccines. These foreign compounds being injected have to go somewhere, they deposit in parts of the body, mimicking the molecules in our joints which is known as molecular mimicry, also in the tissues and the body sees them as foreign compounds and literally starts attacking itself, such as rheumatoid arthritis.

The point is that they are now doing a study because they have made SO many children sick, hospitalized them with the flu and pneumonia. How is this legal?? Are we halting all shots until we get to the bottom of it?

I hear over and over of elderly people, not just children, getting the flu shot and then next thing you know, they have the flu. Odds are they wouldn't have gotten it if they didn't give it to themselves. But we are set up based on fear, being pushed by our doctors.

Formaldehyde, Mercury and Aluminum

As if it's not enough, they also contain Formaldehyde, Mercury and Aluminum. I am not sure if parents do not understand how toxic to human life these substances are, but I can assure you if anybody else was doing this to babies and children, it would not be ok.

Exposure to mercury leads to systemic health problems running the gamut from neurological dysfunction (memory loss, confusion, inability to concentrate) to depression, renal failure, skin troubles and gastrointestinal disturbances. There have actually been links from vaccines to asthma as well as autism. I n German children, 11 percent of those vaccinated reported having ear infections, compared to less than 0.5 percent of unvaccinated children. Similarly, sinusitis was reported in over 32 percent of vaccinated children, while the prevalence in unvaccinated children was less than one percent.

The MMR vaccine is supposed to make you immune to measles, mumps and rubella … yet *77 percent* of the 1,000+ who were sickened with mumps were vaccinated in previous years.

Died At 6 Years Old

We, sadly, had a little girl die in our town, only 6 years old after receiving a flu shot, the next day she was gone. She had nothing wrong with her before she went to the doctor for a 'routine checkup.' I feel that if I didn't put this in my book and if someone who might've seen it would've made a different choice if they had seen it and it saves just one child's life, then I won't worry about the possible people that I pushed away with the facts.

The slightest possibility that I could save a child's life, save an unsuspecting parent from the horrible devastating loss of their loved one meant I had to include this vital lifesaving information. I will include a lot of resources for you too, so you can do your homework.

Only you know what's right for your family, only you can choose. Some parents decide after research to get a few shots and decline the others. But if we just think for a minute, about giving little babies Hep. B as soon as they come out, first of all, if their family has no history of it, I'm pretty sure you only risk exposure during sex or when using drugs and sharing needles, right?

Then why would a newborn need that shot? Quite sure they're not going to be having sex or doing drugs 'til at least they can walk, right?

If immunizations are chosen, they can be administered when the child is older over a period of time instead of putting such a strain on your child's immune system. If given when they're older around the age of 7 or older, then their immune system should be stronger than when they're younger.

Vaccine Injured

Have you ever heard the term 'vaccine injured?' When they pay them off for the destruction of their loved one's life, it s called an 'award.' These are the families who have received billions from Big Pharma for either permanently disabling their babies or worse. If you believe these vaccines are so safe, I'm sure they'd have a different story to tell.

Dr. Mercola cites, 'Today, most of the awards go to adults injured by flu shots (64,65,66) while thousands of families whose children have died or suffered catastrophic vaccine injuries are left with nothing but medical bills and shattered lives. Clearly, public health officials do not want to concede that the risks of vaccination for children are far greater than 1 in a million.'

The National Childhood Vaccine Injury Act

As a result of all of the litigation and billions that were being 'awarded' to families monetizing their loved one's disability or death, a law was passed -The National Childhood Vaccine Injury Act- (sounds like it's for children, doesn't it?) eliminating the potential financial liability of vaccine manufacturers acknowledging that vaccine injuries and deaths are real. So, no more suing, know that if your baby is one of those 1 in however many, no more compensation.

All I'm going to say is do your research especially if you have a teenager coming around whose doctor is going to want to inject with the HPV vaccine. They are injecting boys now when it's supposed to be a vaccine for cervical cancer and a freshman boy died after his second round.

Research all of the girls in Columbia, France, Japan who swear they were normal, healthy girls before the vaccine and now they're not, with no compensation or even sympathy in some cases, if you research those poor girls in Columbia whom they insisted were suffering from 'mass hysteria' after the vaccine, instead of having vaccine reactions, it might make you cry, I did. These are our children we are talking about.

In other countries, mothers are standing up for their babies and joining together protesting this cruel practice. Specifically, in Ireland, they are rising up, making noise and getting the attention of the media, getting their messages out there. When you take your baby in for a check-up, you want to come home with the same child you left with and unfortunately for these parents of vaccine-injured children, there's no going back, their children will never be the same again.

Watching them is heartbreaking and all of them say, they thought it was safe and wish they had known. This is why I was obligated to include this as my tribute to them from one parent to another parent. The worst part is that some who actually lost their babies had reservations or questions and were pressured by their doctor. Now they just wish they had researched a little more...

An excellent resource is Robert F. Kennedy, he started an organization called the Children's Health Defense fighting for our children's rights. I would strongly suggest looking him up if this interests you, he is a wealth of knowledge.

Some useful links:

https://www.littlemountainhomeopathy.com/how-to-prevent-vaccine-injury

http://tenpennyimc.com/2012/11/26/flu-vaccine-isnot-a-good-idea-for-your-child/

https://www.youtube.com/watch?v=fA1NfaMuEx

https://www.youtube.com/watch?v=xEcYQydhY9E#action=share

https://articles.mercola.com/sites/articles/archive/2011/11/0
1/more-parentswaking-up-to-vaccine-dangers.aspx
https://vaccines.mercola.com/

https://www.youtube.com/watch?v=XIRXxEYnkxA

https://www.youtube.com/channel/UCnZ_o5cpwkHJuEYjPt
M0j5A

https://www.hrsa.gov/vaccinecompensation/about/in-
dex.html

https://www.fairwarning.org/2018/12/vaccine-court-pays-bil-
lions/

Viruses

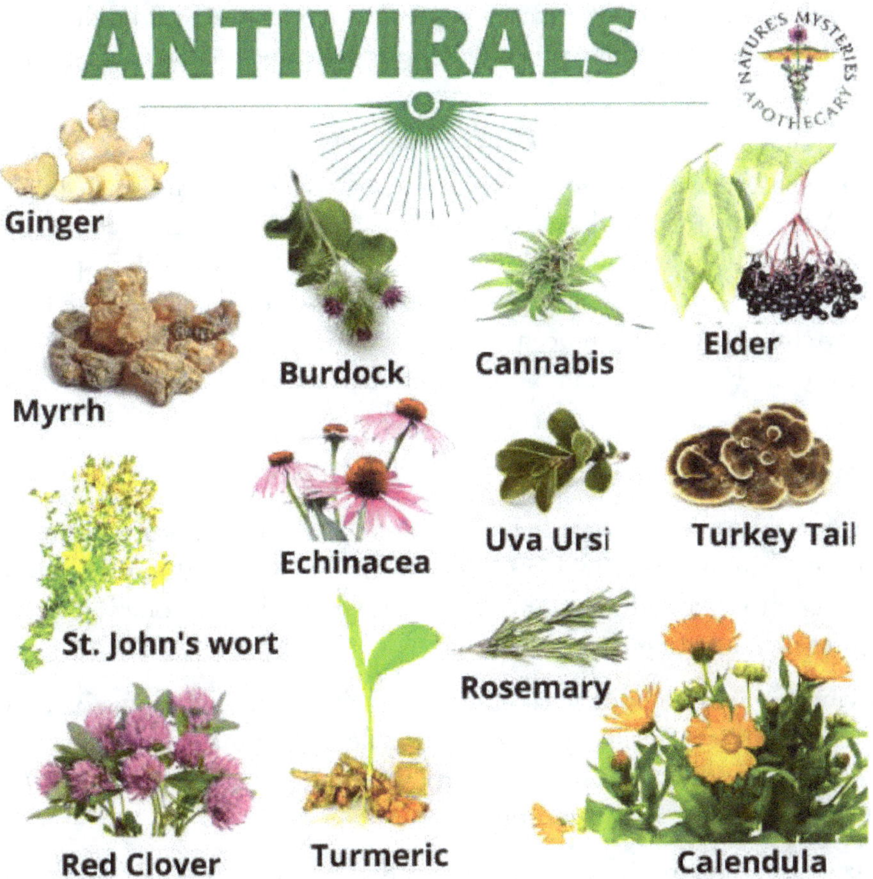

These plants should be in your first line of defense when going up against a virus. The way that disease works in the body depends on whether it's viral, bacterial, etc. Viral infections cannot be addressed with antibiotics. For children suffering from a virus, being given an antibiotic, which is annihilating all of the friendly bacteria in their gut, where 80% of their immune system lies, just means that you actually improved the conditions for the pathogen to grow, lessening the body's ability to fight it off, naturally.

We actually know now that the effects of antibiotics can be devastating to the immune system and should only be used as a last resort. If an individual has been on antibiotics more than two times it is said that they should take supplemental probiotics to increase the gut flora for a period of up to two years!

The way that a virus works in the body is not commonly known. Viruses such as HIV have incomplete DNA and are trying to steal some of your DNA to make their molecule complete. Eventually, the cell becomes depleted and 'bleached out.' When this occurs, the cell explodes, spewing out the contents of the virus, spreading the disease. But there have been many children who have been given antibiotics to treat a viral infection, unfortunately, not only inhibiting but destroying the child's immune system.

Natural Antibiotics

Some folks are not aware that there are natural antibiotics that are an excellent alternative with the same effectiveness rate without risking it turning into a 'superbug' immune to their antibiotics. No one is a better fighter than a strong immune system.

Giving your child's body what it needs to fight and not inhibiting or eliminating its function is like giving them a shield. And that's not to say that they might not come down with something, kids get sick, but it's HOW sick they get that is the question.

I have seen children put on antibiotics that don't do anything so they'll put them on another round. But all the time, I just knew that if that poor child were given some herbs, they would get better, without a doubt, whatever the cause of illness. Herbs restore balance to your child's body on many levels. All the while, ensuring proper nutrition and eliminating sugar and artificial colors, flavors, etc. that can inhibit immune function will increase recovery time.

Forest Bathing

Spend some time in the woods, if you can. Research done in Japan now proves that 'forest bathing' (spending time in the forest) increases your white blood cells known as natural killer cells (NK). After 3 days in the forest, those NK levels rose by 50%!!! These are the white blood cells that attack and fight infections and tumor cells. And perhaps the best part? This increase lasted for 30 days! Fascinating, huh?

Here is a link if you'd like to learn more:

https://www.ncbi.nlm.nih.gov/pmc/articles/PMC2793341/

So take them for a walk in the woods, better yet, go camping! Or you can crank the tunes up and have a Dance Party!

Dance Party

Music not only raises your child's vibration but actually increases their immune system function according to a study done in Leipzig Germany. This study found that under an hour of upbeat dance music raised the level of antibodies in the participants. As well as immunoglobulin A levels (which are the body's first line of defense when encountering pathogens) not only that, stress hormone levels such as cortisol decreased as well, which translates into less inflammation of whatever kind that the body is suffering from.

Earthing

Basically, just placing your feet on the Earth and absorbing the electromagnetic current running through the soles of your feet can not only induce a sense of well-being, but can reduce cortisol levels. Now that we understand that we are made of electricity, frequencies and vibrations, it makes sense that feeling the Earth under our bare feet is grounding.

By coming in direct contact with Mother Earth's surface, not only providing us with food, water, fresh air, but we actually receive a charge of energy from deep within. Knowing that the Earth has an electrical current running through it, with ley lines and specific courses that the energy of the Earth's circuits run through, only makes sense that we would feel depleted if we didn't connect with it.

Seasonal Affective Disorder

This would also explain Seasonal Affective Disorder. This disorder makes us feel sick from a lack of Sun, vitamin D, full-spectrum light and feeling our feet sink into grass, or sand, or a nearby stream. We actually require this transference of energy with the natural world to feel our best.

It is thought that many of the Ancient Sacred Sites that are known but misunderstood by people today are built on these ley lines. So, once again, not only did our ancestors know the curative powers of plants way before their time, but they also understood healing concepts about energy that we are only beginning to grasp.

Natural Ways to Improve Immune Function

Forest Bathing –
Echinacea –
Manuka Honey –
Colloidal Silver (Sovereign Silver) –
CBD Oil –

Not Always Better

It doesn't always mean that it is better for your child because you don't see the symptoms anymore, bringing down a fever might make you feel better because your child doesn't look so hot, but might not be the best thing for your child's body. A fever is one of the ways that the body tries to fight off an invader, by making the temperature so hot that it burns it out.

While this can be uncomfortable for your child, there are things that you can do to make them more comfortable, while allowing the body to perform its natural function and to avoid the possibility of creating a situation where your child will be more likely to acquire illnesses throughout their life.

Every time your child gets sick and their body fights it off naturally, without any kind of pharmaceutical assistance, it is stronger for it. Now, this doesn't mean that we want to let our children suffer, by any means, teas can be administered, compresses can be applied to the forehead and chest, essential oils can be rubbed on their feet and within hours you will see improvement.

That is if sugar is eliminated and artificial flavors, colors, preservatives, processed foods, uncomfortable situations, as well. All of the contributing factors that lead to insufficient immune function.

Why Children Get Sick

Sometimes children get sick as a result of their environment. Sometimes perhaps, to be noticed by their parents who will not or cannot slow down to give them attention, unless they're sick. We now know that emotions can cause disease in the body so if a child is going through a stressful time such as divorce, loss of a loved one, moving away from family, substance abuse in the family or sexual abuse, there are many conditions that can contribute to a child not feeling well even if it seems like they are being fed, kept warm and taken care of. With so many soul nourishing, immune-boosting herbs available, your child will feel better in no time!

My Go-Tos for Immune Boosting

- **Echinacea/Goldenseal** combinations are great

- **Astragalus** potent immune booster

- **Green Tea** (I like Yogi brand, you can get a decaffeinated version)

- **Nettle** the most nutritious plant in the plant kingdom, dries up mucus

- **Chamomile** a little can be added to calm them down and settle their little nerves and add a sweet flavor

- **Manuka Honey (for children over 1 year of age)** Under 1-year-old, possible botulism poisoning from bacteria found in the honey that the tender immune system cannot process until after 1 year of age. Happens rarely but not worth risking

- **Colloidal Silver** by Sovereign Silver (the only company that I would use)

- **CBD Oil** responsible for maintaining cellular homeostasis, start with 2 drops in the morning and 2 drops and night for three days

Colloidal Silver (by Sovereign Silver only)

Did I say silver? Yes. For immune-boosting? Yes. Antibiotic, antiviral, anti-bacterial, anti-fungal, kills everything in a test tube, one of your best friends! Throughout your life, not just limited to children.

There have been records from many ancient civilizations such as the Egyptians, Romans, Greeks and Phoenicians utilizing the healing potential of silver. Phoenicians actually stored their water, wine and vinegar in silver bottles aware of its antimicrobial possessing powers.

For 6,000 years, it has been a welcome addition to Herbal Apothecaries, as a crucial aid in restoring health, Hippocrates used it for wound care.

Silver nitrate was used in the 1800s to treat wounds and skin ulcers.

Before refrigeration, in the Old West, a silver coin might be tossed in a bottle of milk or water because it could prevent the growth of algae, bacteria, fungi, etc.

During the Civil War, it was used to combat syphilis.

You might have heard of putting Silver nitrate in babies' eyes after they were born?

In the 1890s, colloidal silver was discovered and recorded as being administered as the immune booster of choice; by the 1930s, it was used in World War 1 to address wounds and infections.

The Apollo spacecraft approved the use of silver ions to kill bacteria in their water and NASA approved a silver-based water purification system for the International Space Station.

Silver use declined with the emergence of antibiotics, but is still used in burn centers. They have put it in a creme called Sulfadiazine blended with some petrochemicals such as white petrolatum, propylene glycol and water with methylparaben, of course!

Silver is an element found in medicinal and edible mushrooms, mammalian milk, whole grains, seawater, spring water and tap water. Used over time as a welcome aid in restoring health merely containing just nanoparticles of silver suspended in water.

All colloidal silvers are not the same; that is, they are not all created alike. I feel like what I'm about to say is going to make you not want to use it, but I have used it safely for 30 years, it's like anything else, used as directed, you're fine.

So, if the particles are not small enough and with extended use, it can make your skin actually take on a green or grey hue. This is why I said I wouldn't use any companies other than Sovereign Silver. None of us have any tint or greenish greyish hue to our skin!

Dose:
Read the label and dose accordingly. For children, usually one dropper is adequate. After administering colloidal silver alternating with Echinacea, I usually did not have to use it for more than **3 days, 5 days tops, and that is using it 3 to 4 times a day**. This dose is completely safe.

People use pharmaceuticals all of the time willing to risk a stroke or a heart attack and think nothing of it. The only way that you'd experience any side effects from colloidal silver would be if you didn't use it as directed. Pharmaceuticals result in side effects not only if used as directed, if they are used at all, it's a possibility.

Excellent Uses:

- **Nasal infections**: Drop a couple drops directly in the nose, use for 10 days

- **Pneumonia, congestion or bronchitis**: Excellent treatment for pneumonia when taken internally as an alternative to conventional treatments. Antibiotics are often being administered meaning as we said above that if the pneumonia is viral in nature will not be effective. The most effective method to get the colloidal silver into the lungs is to use a nebulizer, breathing it in allowing it to come into direct contact with the germs invading the lungs.

Generally, use 1 teaspoon approximately three times a day for 10 to 15 minutes.

- **Pink Eye**: Drop a couple drops in eye a few times a day

- **Ear Infection**: Drop a couple drops in ear a few times a day

- **Ringworm**: Drop a few drops directly a few times a day or soak a cotton ball and hold on there for 5 min. three times a day

- **Antiseptic**: Excellent for wound care, scrapes, cuts, etc. Doesn't sting like Bactine.

- **Rashes**: Take internally and externally, internally follow directions on bottle depending on age and apply externally as compress with soaked cotton balls.

Rash

When a child experiences a rash, it is the body's way to remove some kind of toxins that it has come in contact with. Our skin is one of our filters, our largest organ, absorbing 60% of whatever we apply to it, the body tries to eliminate toxins through the skin. Sweating is a way that our body removes toxins.

If a child experiences a rash and we give them Benadryl, which stops the body's natural reaction of trying to remove whatever it is that is creating imbalance within the system, it doesn't remove whatever was creating the imbalance in the system, it just removes your child's natural ability to remove whatever was causing the imbalance in their system.

That is why the importance of not removing symptoms cannot be stressed enough especially if it's just being done to make the parents feel better. By applying compresses to the rash with healing herbs that enable all of the bodies eliminating processes to perform their duty while making your child feel comfortable at the same time, is the balance that is the goal.

A healing ointment with either Calendula oil or a salve made with Calendula flowers, Lavender, Rose, St. John's wort, can be applied along with some herbs that have antibacterial and antifungal properties to help disinfect the area and keep it free of bacteria and germs.

Herbs that are immune-boosting can be added to this tea blend to assist the body in not only eliminating toxins but building the immune system, as well. Make sure to keep the area dry, moist conditions can improve the growth of bacteria.

Juice Was Too Acidic

When my girls were little I could actually see by the acidity of their urine when they would drink orange juice because their bottoms would start getting red or a rash even, would show up. As babies and toddlers, they couldn't drink any kind of super acidic drinks such as pineapple juice, orange juice, grapefruit juice, etc. if I wanted to give them any other kind of juice I would have to water it down 3 to 1 being three parts water one part juice. And then they could drink it and have it not create redness and soreness on their bottoms.

As a result, I just watered down all juices before giving it to them, to reduce the natural sugar intake as well as reduce the level of acidity in the drink.

Trace It Back

If parents do not pay attention to what they feed their little ones and try to associate it when they see an imbalance in their child's system or behavior, by trying to trace it back to what could have caused it, if it was something new that has been introduced into the child's environment as an example.

And not just go to a pediatrician hoping for a prescription while never exploring the possibilities of why or what created the imbalance stemming within their child's system, then further imbalance and damage can be created by the use of improperly prescribed medications that are given unnecessarily especially when natural medicine could be administered that would not only help the body process whatever is trying to be eliminated or indicated but can actually build it, strengthen it and increase the level of white blood cell production and other fighter T cells that increase the likelihood of health and longevity for your child.

When your child is given compounds that they cannot process they can accumulate in their system which can eventually create such an imbalance that the proper levels of other important compounds are minimized because of a lack of space, we need to ask ourselves is this really medicine.

Sugar can fit into receptors taking up space where vital messages from neurotransmitters are supposed to be - not allowing messages from the body to get through creating further imbalances because the necessary hormones are either not being produced or are being suppressed because the brain's messages are not getting through.

Caffeine

Some pharmaceutical medications even have caffeine in them, among other chemicals that are not good for children and can increase hyperactivity as well. As we know sugar can cause hyperactivity, as well as other food additives. If this occurs, the child is usually given some kind of medication to calm them down or stop them from being so hyper when it's actually the food that they are consuming that is creating this kind of hyperactivity.

School lunches are full of processed agents, sugar, artificial flavors and preservatives and other chemicals that a child should never come in contact with, much less eat. Some of which are even known to be carcinogenic to men and yet they're being served to our children on a daily basis under the cloak labeled food.

I have seen this time and again, when my daughters were young, I was a Creative Movement teacher at seven different after school programs and two different libraries. Because I was coming in after school, a lot of the children were eating snacks in the after school program, many of the snacks were brightly colored and completely toxic and about 15 minutes after the children had snack time, complete chaos would ensue.

The children would be yelled at, corrected, punished, one school went so far as to make assigned seating during the after school program, which basically was a result of how toxic their snacks were.

The children were not bad students, I never had any problems when we were in class, but the way that the adults talked to them and the food they were being fed was just such a sorry sight to behold and actually pained my heart to watch.

Kids are in a structured environment for 8+ hours a day, and for those children who have to stay in school until 5 PM, to still be in such a structured, tight, oppressive environment for so many hours out of their day, even when it's in the afterschool program, is not creating the kind of world that I want to see.

Sugary Sweet

If everything we give our children is sugary and sweet, the potential of ruining their taste buds is risked. So that when they taste real food, it's not sweet enough and then they won't want to eat it. I didn't need to add any honey to my daughter's tea blends. They would drink them just as they were and one of my daughters wouldn't drink it with honey because it was too sweet for her.

Most children would drink tea without any added sugar, try it that way first, if you have to add some honey you can. If it's for a sore throat or cough, then you actually want to add the honey, but I wouldn't make a habit of it in general, so that your child will drink tea even if there's no sweetener added.

Tainted Taste Buds

Some children's taste buds get so tainted that they try to say they aren't going to eat anything but Cheetos and Chicken Nuggets. I've actually encountered parents who told me, "That's all they eat…"

First of all, if they are small, we are in charge of what they eat, teenagers being more of a challenge. But my suggestion is to tell children that after they eat their food, they can have something that they'd like, 'a treat' so to speak.

And if it's that that they are offered: nothing or offered something that they like to eat after they finish their food and it has digested, every time, my girls would eat their food, so that they could have the treat. There wasn't always a treat offered, but that's how it worked when there was.

They also couldn't have it as soon as they were done, they had to wait 10-15 minutes for their food to digest a little bit. They knew this, they might roll their eyes when I said it, but they knew it was coming and so does my grandson.

Whole Grains, Fruits and Vegetables

I have found that if you feed children good food such as fruits and vegetables, whole grains from the very beginning, they enjoy them. And this didn't only work with my daughters, it is true with my 3 grandsons as well who will eat vegetables that other children turn their nose up to.

Don't get me wrong, they have veggies that are not their favorite, but they have plenty of others that they enjoy. Everyone's taste buds are not the same. As an example, one grandson loves peas, one loves radishes and the other loves broccoli and all of them absolutely adore avocados!

Childhood Obesity Rate

The childhood obesity rate and childhood diseases that children never had before, are a direct result of not only our SAD- Standard American Diet, but also a result of the explosion of technology and the lack of general exercise that children would normally experience on a daily basis.

Children and Cellphones

Nowadays, as soon as many children open their eyes, they're either handed a phone, or go into a room where there is a TV on, or are in the car where there's a screen on the back of their parents' seat, or even worse, have their own cell phone. The studies and the findings on these are shocking when considered how damaging a cell phone could be to a young child's developing brain.

The World Health Organization published conclusive evidence-based research that cell phones increase the rate of brain cancer. Russia has banned the use of all WiFi and cell phones in elementary schools, recently, in response to the growing body of evidence that these waves are harmful to young children's brains and reproductive organs. According to Robert F. Kennedy, in 2013, Israel banned WiFi in kindergartens and limited its use in elementary schools.

Knowing the risks or even the possibility of this should increase our understanding of the disservice we are doing to our children when we give them not only their own cell phone or hand them our cell phone, but we are actually damaging their brains.

Remember what we said about other countries paying for their citizens health care? I'm not going to go into detail in this book, but I will say

look up the effects of 5G from a reputable source and they are frightening.

Limit EMFs and Cell Phone Exposure

From our earlier chapters, learning about vibrations, frequencies, electromagnetic fields, and the effects of these on the human body and the interference it causes and the likeliness of disease when this happens, we
wouldn't want to blame ourselves in the end if something happened to
our children as a result of our actions that could have been avoided.

Children are very sensitive to subtle energies and their developing cells
are fragile and can be easily damaged by harmful emissions emanating
from our electronics. WiFi devices, Bluetooth devices, Xboxes, laptops,
computers, etc., these electromagnetic imbalances can begin on an energetic level and if ignored can begin to create imbalances within the physical body.

As we said Russia and now others such as France, Italy, Belgium, Spain,
Israel and Australia have begun taking actions to eliminate or reduce Wi-
Fi and cell phones in schools. As far back as 2015 the Environmental
Health Trust (EHT) issued the following release:

'Teton Village, WY —(SBWIRE) —09/22/2015 —

As of this fall, Israel and Italy are officially recommending schools reduce
children's exposures to wireless radiation. The Israeli Ministry of Health
has initiated a major public awareness effort to reduce wireless and electromagnetic radiation exposures to children. In similar action, the Italian
State Parliament of South Tyrol voted to allow the application of the
precautionary principle to replace existing wireless networks whenever
possible with wired networks or those that emit less radiation.

The Israeli Ministry of Health (MoH) recommendations are published in
the Environmental Health in Israel Report 2014 which states that "Pre-
cautions should be strictly enforced with regard to children, who are
more sensitive to developing cancer. "The Report makes the following
points: Cell Phones: "The MoH recommends sensible use of cellular and

wireless technology, including: considering alternatives like landline telephones" MoH recommendations include: use a speaker or hands-free phone accessory or (non-wireless) personal earphone in order to distance the telephone from the body, reduce the amount and duration of calls, and in areas of weak reception reduce calls because of higher radiation. Children: MoH recommends: "refraining from installing the base of wireless phones in a bedroom, work room, or children's room." Schools: Levels of non-ionizing radiation were measured in 25 schools nationwide and "based on these findings, the MoEP recommends that students remain at a distance of at least 1.5 meters from electrical cabinets and that use of wireless communication networks in schools be reduced.

Reduce Exposure in Cars: The MoH recommends not using cellphones in closed places like cars or elevators, buses, and trains unless there is an external antenna "due to amplified radiation in such places." "When driving, a hands-free device should be used for calls.

It is recommended to install an antenna outside the vehicle and to use a line connection between the telephone and the speaker as opposed to using Bluetooth.

Research: Previous research findings in Israel "clearly indicated a link between cellphone use for more than 10 years and the development of tumors in the salivary glands." Israel is currently a partner in two additional international studies: (1) MOBI-Kids, a multi-center study involving experts from 16 countries who are examining potential associations between use of communication devices and other environmental factors and risk of brain tumors, and (2) the GERoNiMO (Generalised EMF Research using Novel Methods) project, which uses an integrated approach and expertise from 13 countries to further the state of knowledge on EMF and health.'

It is not opinion or belief that cell phones are detrimental to children's developing brains, this is now fact proven by research.

EMF Protection

If you are in a place where you have no choice and there are towers around you that you have no control over, there are actions you can implement to intervene in the damage to your cells. There are materials that can neutralize the harmful frequencies emanating from these towers and devices so that they are not harmful.

Briefly, I'd recommend that you research Shungite, it is a mineral from Russia with a rare molecular composition and it has the ability to neutralize these dangerous frequencies. Referred to as The Stone Of Life. It actually has antioxidant properties which react with EMF's (electromagnetic field) harmonizing them.

EMF Blues is a business that sells protection from EMF's and 5G, not only neutralizing them but harmonizing them. There are a lot of companies out there proclaiming a lot of things, but in my research, EMF Blues panned out to be the most reputable.

I've had their cell phone tabs on my cell phone since I started using one. They also have Crystal Catalyst Resonators that you can put on your computers, WiFi routers, etc.

Knowing that we are energetic beings and that every living cell in our body is vibrating at its own frequency makes it easy to understand what kind of detrimental health effects can result from an interference with the vibration of our frequency.

Fever

A child having a fever is a natural process that their bodies needs to go through, if it gets up to be 104, then a physician might recommend something else being administered. We always used the Homeopathic Remedy, Belladonna, with great success! I had three babies in five years and they definitely experienced every day, childhood illnesses that children experience throughout their childhood.

They never received Tylenol as an option for making them feel better. Never, in their whole life did they ever take Children's Tylenol or Benadryl or any other over-the-counter drugs. And we never ended up in the emergency room because their fevers spiked.

Their fevers did get high, but when they started soaring I would give them Belladonna and it would bring it back down, every time the same with my grandson when he was sick and at my house.

At the first sign or indication that one of my girls was under the weather or not feeling themselves, low energy, etc. I would reach for the Echinacea. This was a tincture that I made from our Echinacea plants that we grew. But one from the health food store would work as well as long as organic standards are ensured. I would try to get one from a local Herbalist who you trust.

Echinacea Dose

1 dropperful of tincture
1 cup of water
Three times a day as needed until symptoms start improving.
This can be repeated for 2 weeks.
By then the child should be better. If further immune boosting is required, regimen can be repeated after a 2 week lapse is up.

If there is a fever presenting and the child starts crying or getting very uncomfortable, I'd recommend the following:

Belladonna Homeopathic

6x or 6c, 30x or 30c whichever you can find.

Dose:

2-4 pellets under the tongue.

Note: Do not touch Homeopathic Remedies with your fingers as the oils on your fingers can affect absorption.

Just have your little one tilt their head back and put the cap by their open mouth tilting it, so the pellets fall under their tongue.

If symptoms are less severe:
1-2 pellets under the tongue

More severe symptoms
4 pellets, repeat three times a day.
If a high fever is present, Homeopathic doses can be repeated every 15 minutes until the condition is stable.

It is not recommended that any strong herbs, medications or other compounds such as toothpaste that could affect the remedy be given within 15 minutes of administration. Take 30 minutes outside of meals. Because absorption takes place through the membranes in the mouth, contents of the stomach do not have any effect.

Dr. Maria Montessori Methods for Behavioral Issues

When my girls were young, I became a Montessori teacher for 3-9-year-olds and opened the Wildflower Montessori School. Dr. Maria Montessori was the first woman doctor in Italy. She actually contributed to the end of child labor there as well. She performed years of research on children, mostly just observing them.

As I learned of her teaching method, it resonated with every cell in my body, sharing many of her beliefs and observations of children from homeschooling and raising my daughters.

She worked with intellectually disabled children that they called names and kind of disregarded at this point in time. Dr. Montessori believing children to be the 'lost citizens,' structured an environment for them with 'Montessori Materials' a series of Didactic 'hands on' teaching materials that the children 'played' with, but the whole time they were learning different math concepts, reading, vocabulary, science, etc. all under the pretense of 'playing.'

These intellectually disabled children started scoring higher on tests than the 'normal' children. So they started wondering what she was doing and many schools have implemented not only her teaching materials but her methods as well, such as not interrupting children when they are working and observing a 3 hour work period to name a few.

Her schools are all over the world and her methods are worth investigating as a parent or any kind of child care provider. Utilizing her techniques with children will make your life 100% easier! I have included some of our combined recommendations that I used. I would give parents these recommendations as part of a workshop that I taught and hopefully they will make your life as a parent a little easier:

Recommendations for Making Life with Children Easier:

- Eye level when speaking

- Lost citizen: make sure to have furniture their size such as small tables and chairs to work at

- Dignity: don't call them out if they do something wrong, explaining why, instead of punishment and ostracizing them so they can retain their dignity

- Choices: Say, "Do you want me to?" or, "Can you do it yourself?" A lot of parents use this one.

- Very literal – avoid sarcasm

- Show first, then tell: children's brains cannot comprehend both at the same time

- Do not show anger or frustration: take a deep breath, count to five, take a break, come back

- Gentle reminders: Say, "Let's not do that right now," instead of "Stop it!" Or you could say, "Remember, I asked if you could…" (do whatever it is you want them to do). If a small child is doing something that you don't want them to do, don't say, "Stop it, don't do that," and leave it at that. Say instead, "Why don't you come and do this?" You might explain what you don't want, but focusing on and directing their attention towards what you want them to do will always end with more success, than if you don't, they need that direction.

- No direct references: Say, "Let's not do that," or "Let's come over here and look at this."

- Concentration: deep, uninterrupted – when children are in deep concentration, if they are not interrupted, they grow a little every time.

- 5 minute warning: mentally prepare themself by giving them the time to organize their last 5 minutes. Instead of saying, "Let's go," when they are right in the middle of something, you wouldn't like it if someone did that to you.

- Sensitive period for order: 3-to-6-year-olds find comfort in organization and knowing where things go, shelves are better than a toy box.

- Mirror feelings: so many emotions, sometimes repeating back what we hear them say helps them move on just to know someone understood how they were feeling.

- Understand feelings: sympathy, it's rough being small and being told what to do, not that they can do what they want but we can be compassionate and caring when we say no. Instead of, "No, we're not getting ice cream."

You could say, "I understand that you'd like some now and I would too, actually, but we have to eat our food first and then maybe later we can get some."

A lot of times, they never even remember to ask for whatever it was that they saw that they wanted at the instant and instead of making them cry and saying, "No," we can just put it off and say, "Yea, maybe later."

Avoid conflict, often that will be enough for them to move on, but if you said, "Not a chance," they'd argue, cry and get themselves into trouble. Why not just avoid that all together?

- Few words: more is less, don't over explain.

- No correction: show how, not how not to, if it's not something drastic and they don't do it right, you don't need to say, "Not like that."

By you showing them the right way, they will notice that they are not doing it right, they have a great sense of detail. Oftentimes if you try to correct them, they say, "I can't do it."

- Praise effort: children need attention, if the way they get it from you is by doing stuff they know you don't want them to do, then they will do it. If they get praised when they act right, they will do their best to get that praise.

- Nothing perfect: try not to say, "That's perfect." If you don't say it next time, they'll always be thinking it's not good enough. Just tell them what you like about it.

- "Ok, Mama" – I always made my girls say this after I told them something so I knew they heard me and couldn't say later, "I didn't hear you."

- Role model: I think this one speaks for itself.

- Independence in situations: makes them feel useful when they help, let them help you do daily household chores.

- Don't pass on your opinion: if you say you don't like a food, most likely they will too. Keep your opinions to yourself, let them develop their own personality.

- Outdoors: best place

- Turn off the TV: ADHD

- Don't help unless asked: don't help without asking, let them try even if it takes them 50 tries, that's how they learn.

- RELAX: don't rush them: they are learning motion - not completing a task.

- Rationalize: does that sound nice or does this sound nicer? My girls would always agree it sounded better to say it nice.

- Can you open your heart to your friend … (and let them …)

- "Because I love you and I don't want you to get hurt is why I don't want you to do this." Instead of, "Because I said so!"

- "You're such a good listener!" – Just keep telling them that and they'll want to keep hearing it.

- Positive affirmations: you're so nice, so generous, so smart, kind, loving, gentle, etc. (every one you can think of). I was doing this with my grandson one time and he said, "You forgot generous," when he was like 5 years old, so sweet!

- Pet kitty nice (by showing them how to pet a cat or dog) – stroke face and say, "be nice" as you rub their hand on your face.

- Tell them what you expect, what to do, not what not to do - guidance.

- Don't condemn, curse: "This could happen." "I know you don't want to," instead of, "You're going to break your neck!"

- Consequences: this way they learn if I do this, this happens, but if I do that, this happens.

- Discuss possible outcomes

- Choose battles

- Cooperative games – see **www.familypastimes.com** – games don't always have to be competitive, sometimes it's nice to play games where you are actually working cooperatively towards the same goal, helping each other out. We had a number of these in my Montessori School and the children loved them. The above website has some of those games.

One of my favorite books is, *The Secret of Childhood* by Dr. Montessori and another one is, *You Are Your Child's First Teacher*, by Rahima Baldwin Dancy. I would highly recommend them.

Proper Nutrition

Because children's bodies are still developing and continuing to change, utilizing large amounts of energy for all of this growing, the importance of giving them the proper nutrition for optimum growth cannot be stressed enough.

Feeding children highly processed high fructose corn syrup laden cereals for breakfast and then choosing hormone induced, nitrate filled meats for lunch, with processed chicken nuggets covered in genetically modified wheat and corn with chickens that were injected with hormones to make them reach 20 pounds in a short amount of time that lived in a tiny cage where they couldn't even lift their wings so they would mature quickly increasing the chicken industries yields, could be resulting in our children getting sick.

It is not hard to figure out where these diseases stem from. The farther we move away from natural foods for our children, the closer we will come to increasing the levels of disease in our children.

A good children's multivitamin such as from New Chapter, is always a good choice to ensure proper nutrition. So if one day they don't eat as much of their veggies as you wish, you have the comfort of knowing that their nutritional needs were at least met with the vitamin. In this case a whole food-based, organic multivitamin would be the only choice.

Our Grandmother's Choices

It is said that the quality of our health can be traced back to our grandmother's choices. In making better choices for ourselves, we are not only increasing our personal longevity, but also the quality of our future generations' immune systems and abilities to fight off disease.

Knowing this, that it is our choices as women, as to the outcome and health of our future generations puts a responsibility in our hands to not only make the important, life-sustaining, health improving choices, but to educate our children to do the same for the preservation of ourselves and our children to come.

By choosing to grow organic gardens, by choosing to feed organic food to our families, by choosing to keep our water systems clean, by choosing to only use biodegradable cleaning products, by choosing to only use organic personal care products, by choosing to make the conscious, sometimes less convenient, but always making a larger impact decision, we can improve not only the health of our children and our future generations, but the health of the planet.

Teach Your Children

What we are lacking in ourselves, we can make up for by teaching our children the right way, the way that is perhaps less traveled, the right way doesn't always mean the popular way.

Sometimes, doing it the right way might not be understood by those around us, but know that just by you choosing what's best ripples out in ways that you sometimes will be aware of and others you will know nothing of, but will feel the repercussions of those ripples when they come back to you.

What's right isn't always popular.

What's popular isn't always right…

My First Aid Kit :

- **Rescue Remedy Bach Flower Remedy**

- **Arnica Homeopathic 6x or 6c**

- **Belladonna 30c or 30x**

- **CBD Oil**

- **Weleda Diaper Rash Crème**

- **Band-aids**

- **Ledum Homeopathic** (instead of a tetanus shot, I carried this around so that if they stepped on a rusty nail, I could give them this great alternative)

Herbs for Children ~

- **Chamomile**

- **Elderberry**

- **Echinacea**

- **Hemp**

- **Calendula**

- **Nettle**

- **Arnica (Homeopathic remedy)**

This illustrates the best choices when considering which herbs to choose for your children:

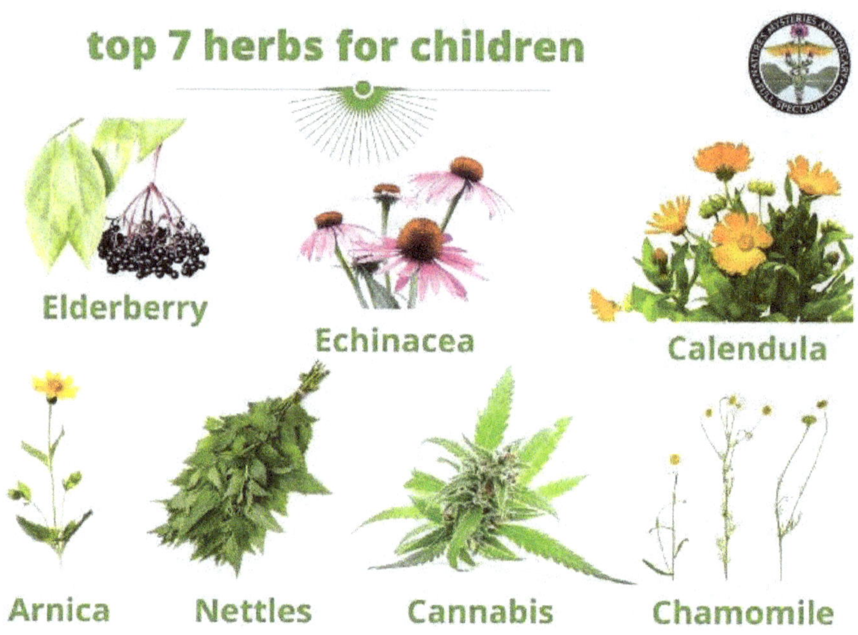

When my daughters were little, CBD was not a remedy that was even an option in the treatment of children. In fact, using Hemp with children would have definitely gotten you arrested!

Children and Hemp

However, now we know what a safe and effective alternative the Hemp plant is for children and how it would be one of our top choices in the treatment of our children. Being one of the safest remedies available offered to parents.

Most medicinal plants are good for children but some are considered unsafe under specific ages. Hemp is not one of those plants, it is actually used on six week old babies. Mother's breast milk contains cannabinoids. Our bodies produce cannabinoids.

With no threat of overdosing, and the versatile nature of the plant, it can be used for relieving the majority of maladies. Considering that it brings the body back into a state of homeostasis (which is balance on all levels from temperature, glucose, appetite, if you have too much of one hormone it will decrease it, not enough of one, it will increase it and it is the only substance on the planet that we know of that we have these receptors for) it is an ideal treatment for alleviating symptoms in a safe effective way.

As we discussed, pharmaceutical medications have never been tested on children as that would be unethical, and we know that we have no receptors for pharmaceutical medications in our bodies, and we are aware of the fact that there is no condition or disease that is due to a lack of pharmaceutical medications.

But knowing that we do have receptors all throughout our bodies for the Hemp plant means that it is a much more viable option for our children due to its safety. Knowing that there are many conditions that are due to an Endocannabinoid deficiency that could be relieved with daily use of the Hemp plant validates its use for children as well.

This sacred plant has alleviated seizure disorders in children when either ingested or vaped. I formulate a CBD infused roll-on gem essence that has been reported to stop seizures in a patient's niece who has Rett's syndrome.

She bought the roll-on for her migraines and one day her niece started having a seizure. They have a heavy-duty pharmaceutical medication that they give her when she has a seizure, but try not to give it to her, but if she seizes for more than four minutes then it is the only option.

On this particular day, the woman took her roll-on and applied it to her niece's temples and the seizure stopped. Everyone in the room all looked at each other as if to say, *'did that really just happen?'* She reported that they have found success using the roll-on 9 times out of 10 for her niece's seizures.

If they see that she is starting to have one, they rub it on her and it will stop it from going any further. And if she is mid seizure they can apply it, and it will stop the seizure immediately.

This is a huge accomplishment, as there are no known topical products that inhibit or stop seizures, even in the conventional medicine field. And all it is plant medicine. A blend of carrier oils complemented by essential oils synergistically combined with magnesium chloride and specific gem-stone chips and then Reiki charged to bring relief.

CBD has also been used as an effective treatment in ADHD for children. In comparison with pharmaceutical medications, the children were able to communicate more effectively and were more vocal.

Right before the publishing of Herbs for Children, I formulated a Roll On Gem Essence that is specially formulated for children with an ADHD or autism diagnosis that can be applied to the child's temples and wrists to help improve focus and increase clarity among other things such as bringing their body back into balance internally.

In regard to temperature, glucose, appetite. Remember, I said turn to Mother Nature every time, she won't let you down. (See Hemp Section for complete profile.)

As Hemp is a soil purifier, removing heavy metals and toxins from the soil, ensuring quality and organic standards cannot be stressed enough.

Nausea

While Mint is an excellent choice for upset stomachs, nausea, vomiting, etc., it is very strong if using the essential oil. In a quart of water, only put 2 drops.

Never smell the oil directly out of the bottle or inhale the tea, can cause nasal irritation if tea is too strong or right out of the bottle. Fresh or dried leaves are a great alternative for tea to the essential oil.

Infusion:
1 tsp. dried herb or
6 good sized leaves

1 cup of hot water

Dose:

Let the child sip throughout the day

CBD Oil blocks the vomit impulse in the brain while relieving nausea and any other imbalances the body is experiencing.

Dose: 2-5 drops under tongue of a low dose of CBD or under (or in tea or water). Call a Clinical Cannabinoid Clinician if you're unsure.

Topically: Mix with castor oil or any other carrier oil and rub directly on belly

Cough/Congestion

Children's Cough Syrup:

1 part Echinacea
3 parts Elderberries
2 parts Wild Cherry Bark
1 part Licorice
Read cautions on plants and see if any apply to your child
before adding to syrup

Stir strong infusion into 1 cup honey
For sedative properties-
Add 1½ parts Chamomile
Directions:

- Concocting a syrup, using a very concentrated decoction by combining herb or herbal blend with water using 2 ounces of herbs per quart of water.

- On low heat bring to a simmer partially covered while simmering liquids down to about half the original volume.

- Strain herbs

- Measure liquid then pour back in pot. Each pint of liquid should have one cup of honey added or maple syrup or vegetable glycerin. A one to one ratio of sweetener to liquid is what most recipes call for.

- Warm mixture stirring well over low heat. Keeping it below 110 degrees to not kill beneficial enzymes in the honey.

- Once removed from heat, fruit concentrate for flavor or a couple of drops of essential oil can be added such as Spearmint, Peppermint, Wintergreen, Orange to aid in preserving the syrup or as a relaxant and aid in the cough formula.

- Pour syrup into bottles, store in the refrigerator where it will last for several weeks.

Honey

So good for children, (not under the age of one) not only does the sweet taste bring a smile to their flushed little faces delighting their taste buds, but its antibiotic, antimicrobial, anti-inflammatory properties including promoting restful sleep, make it a go-to when your child is not feeling well and should be considered one of the first allies to turn to complementing any herbal remedy for pretty much any condition.

Honey has been used for ages, as far back as 15,000 years ago, known as a valuable companion to herbal remedies all over the world such as China, Rome, Greece, Assyria, Egypt. Egyptians believed it to contain a miraculous healing compound that would be passed on to whoever ingested it bestowing power, health, purity and longevity in this world, including protection from the next. Proof of this is found in Pharaohs' tombs where unspoiled sealed jars of honey have been found.

Being one of Mother Nature's richest antimicrobial sources. Possessing potent disinfectant qualities, known as 'hygroscopic.'

Hygroscopic

This means that honey's action involves drawing every bit of moisture out of germs, causing them to perish. Germs require moisture as do humans. Studies, in the past, have shown that the most virulent of germs cannot endure 24-100 hours in this golden liquid, typhoid fever and bronchial pneumonia among two that were tested.

Depending on the flowers the nectar was gathered from and the soil conditions, honey's nutrient content includes in varying degrees: iron, manganese, calcium, copper, silica, chlorine, potassium, phosphorus, vitamins present are B, B2, C, thiamine, riboflavin, pantothenic acid, etc.

Raw Honey

Raw, local, unpasteurized honey from a reputable source is always your first choice. With all of its vitamins, minerals and living enzymes alive and present, honey is a potent healer soothing bronchial passages and easing coughs. When I was pregnant with my daughters, I took a tablespoon of raw honey that had royal jelly, bee pollen and propolis in it every day as a vitamin.

Manuka Honey

Manuka honey is made by bees that pollinate the Manuka tree, in New Zealand. Known to cure staph infections and gingivitis, as well as improving digestive issues. Manuka honey is great medicine for any bacteria-related digestive disorder because of its inherent natural antibiotic, antiinflammatory, antibacterial qualities.

Beneficial Treatment for Milia

(Milia are tiny white bumps that arise on skin.)

Mix Manuka honey with cinnamon and let sit on the affected area for 10-15 minutes, rinse off, repeat as needed.

Now known to be an effective treatment against the antibiotic resistant strain of methicillin-resistant Staphylococcus aureus or MRSA. U.K. researchers from Cardiff Metropolitan University have found that compounds within the honey down regulate the most important genes in the MRSA virus.

Honey Loquat

Another honey product I love that we have the bees to thank for is Honey Loquat, an excellent treatment for sore throats or any kind of congestion, difficulty swallowing, coughs, etc. Original recipe dates back to an ancient Chinese herbal formula from the Han Dynasty (25 BCE). It's a premium quality Chinese traditional soothing beverage that is made by Hans Natural that I would highly recommend having in your natural medicine arsenal.

Bach Flower Remedies

Dr. Edward Bach, born in England in 1886, studied medicine at the University College Hospital. He began to develop an interest in Homeopathy; believing that there was another way to heal besides orthodox medicine – utilizing plants.

Understanding that illness is the effect of disharmony between body and mind, at age 43, he left his prestigious Harley St. practice behind to pursue his research into discovering the mysteries of plant medicine.

He began researching and treating patients for free. By 1932, he had devised 12 of his remedies, continuing his urge to find more. He included 19 more remedies into the series before his death leaving behind a healing legacy.

Only being created by dropping flower petals in water and then letting them remain in the Sun so the extracts of the flowers are infused into the water, which is then bottled, leaving subtle energies behind in the water. There are as many Bach Flower Remedies as there are flowers, but for the purpose of this book, we will limit it to two.

Rescue Remedy

I carried Rescue Remedy and Arnica Homeopathic Remedy with me everywhere I went, when around children. Especially when my little ones were teetering a lot while mastering the art of balance. But really, unfortunately, children are getting hurt all of the time, even if they're not learning to walk.

I carried this for my girls' entire childhood, it is great for any kind of trauma, not just physical, but emotional as well. If they experienced something very upsetting or got bad news or someone hurt their feelings...for whatever reason, matters not.

Dose:

Anytime, your child feels out of balance, a few drops under their tongue and in a few moments, they either forget what was wrong and move on or are better able to understand and deal with the stress at hand, in a more productive, calm manner. It always seemed like a longer duration of discomfort was being experienced if I didn't have Rescue Remedy with me. The differences in recovery time were separated by large margins.

Rock Rose Remedy

A blend of five different Bach Flower Remedies that restore a harmonious balance back to the body, replenish vital energy lost, lowering stress levels, calming the nervous system, relaxing muscles and opening your awareness.

Nightmares

Rock Rose was another remedy used by one of my daughters, who experienced horrible nightmares. Which was baffling because she didn't watch any TV or have any comic books with violence in them or any other scary stories coming into her environment. I was with her every day and I know what she was exposed to, for some reason, she just had nightmares.

What I ended up doing was buying a nighttime children's deck of cards with beautiful vintage drawings on them with sweet sayings to be read before bed to help her drift off to sleep with lovely, wondrous visuals and sweet poetry. We already read a book every night but added this to our bedtime ritual.

I also started giving her Rock Rose Bach Flower Remedy before bed and I think the two complemented each other harmoniously because the nightmares ended and they had been going on for a little while.

Since my girls were little, I started formulating a 'Scary Dreams and Creepy Things Go Away' spray. This can be sprayed under the bed, in closets, behind dressers, on the child's pillow, above the bed, etc. A soothing blend that will calm your little one's fears packed with oils to repel any kind of negative energies, surrounding your little one with protection.

'Scary Dreams and Creepy Things Go Away' Spray:

Blend together in a 1or 2 oz glass spray bottle:

Neroli Hydrosol

EO's of:

Chamomile

Rosemary

Lavender

Mix:

1 oz. Hydrosol

1 drop Rosemary

4 drops Lavender

6 drops Chamomile

Diffuse:

Add a few drops of essential oil blend to a diffuser.

Children's Pain

Arnica

If I didn't have this and my girls got hurt, the crying and sadness associated with the trauma lasted 2 to 4 times longer than if I had Arnica with me. This fact is true, through 4 different children, various ages and varying traumas. I observed so many times the duration of discomfort was markedly extended during the times when I didn't have Arnica compared to moments I did.

CBD Oil

This was not an option for children when my girls were little, but now for my grandsons, it is a go-to if anyone bumps their head or falls down, etc. Either a couple of drops under their tongue or some CBD salve not only takes away the pain, lessens their perception of the pain, but they even kind of forget about it, too.

Topical Application of CBD

Topical products are always a great option for children experiencing pain or anxiety as they can apply it inconspicuously and no one needs to know what it is as opposed to taking a couple of drops which would not be allowed in school and other public places. A topical product such as a roll-on can just be applied to the temples and wrists as needed.

Calming Blend
Combine equal parts:
Hempseed oil
Flaxseed oil
Equal drops of essential oils:
Chamomile
Ylang Ylang
Rose enfleurage
CBD oil (between 5-50mg depending on the severity of the condition) ensuring quality is imperative with this herb, only use organic!
Apply as needed to wrists and temples.
This blend would also be great for easing the anxiety of labor.

Yummy Recipes

So obviously using organic ingredients goes without saying, right? If you did have an immune-compromised child, just substitute the chocolate chips for Lily's Stevia Chocolate Chips.

However, as of yet, I am not aware of any powdered sugar that they could have, just refrain from that part of the recipe.

For the Buckeyes, substitute maple syrup or honey for powdered sugar.

Also, honey can be replaced for maple syrup, in any of the recipes being in Vermont, it's my 'go-to.'

CBD can be added to any of these recipes if you're little ones need a little calming or if they are immune-compromised, this is another great way to administer medicine through food. You can experiment with the dose, if you are not too worried about it you can just add 10 to 15 mg of CBD to the batch. If you want to make sure that each serving has a specific amount of CBD in it then you can just drop a couple of drops onto each serving.

My Favorite Smoothie Recipe

Ingredients:
Juice - apple, peach, mango any one or all
Frozen fruit - cherries, blueberries, strawberries, mangoes, peaches
Bananas
Cottage cheese - 2 tbs. per person
Flaxseed oil - 2 tbs. per person

Directions:
Blend cottage cheese and Flaxseed oil in a blender first until creamy, this is crucial as blending them together is where the magic happens, then add your banana, juice, frozen fruit
Blend until desired consistency, if too thin, add more fruit, if too thick, add more juice
Dose:
8 oz. a day, but we like to drink 2 a day, one in the morning and one at night for dessert
Variations:
CBD Oil -a few drops can be added and stirred in
Sometimes I like to put chocolate chips or cacao nibs
Other additions: raspberries, blackberries, grape juice, cherry juice

Nut Butter and Jelly Roll-up

Ingredients:
Whole grain tortilla
Nut Butter (cashew, almond, peanut)
Jelly or Preserves

Directions:
Take a whole grain tortilla and spread nut butter and jelly (cream cheese is optional).

Roll it up part way, lifting the bottom up and folding over continuing rolling.

Butter pan and sauté roll up 'til golden.

Variations:

Almond butter, cashew butter, peanut butter, etc.

Chocolate chips, cacao nibs, sundrops (natural alternative to M&M's) raisins, cranberries, sliced almonds

What else can you think of?

Get creative!

Cream cheese Roll-up

Same recipe as above but replace nut butter with cream cheese.

One Pan Crazy Cake (VEGAN)

What you'll need:

Baking pan
Spoon
Measuring cup

Ingredients:
1 cup flour
1 cup natural sugar
3 tbs. cocoa

1 tbs. baking soda
3 ½ tbs. Safflower oil
1 tbs. vinegar
1 tsp. vanilla
1 cup water

Directions:

Preheat oven to 350 degrees
Oil pan with ½ tsp of Safflower oil
Pour in dry ingredients, mix thoroughly
Make 3 holes, in one put oil, another put vinegar, and the last one put vanilla - do not mix!
Pour water over all of it, mix and place in the oven for 25-30 minutes.
Variations:
Drop chocolate chips on it after cooking for 15-20 minutes.
This recipe can be made into cupcakes, too.
Frosting (option 1)
1 cup cream cheese
½ cup maple syrup
Blend until creamy and sweet

Variations
Add chocolate syrup, chocolate chips, cocoa, cacao nibs, blueberries, raspberries, cherries, strawberries, coconut, sprinkles
(yes, they have organic ones)
Use honey instead of maple syrup
Frosting (option 2)
1 cup powdered sugar (yes, they have organic powdered sugar)
3 tbs. butter or coconut oil

2-3 tbs. maple syrup or hot water as needed

Variations:
Add chocolate syrup, chocolate chips, cocoa, cacao nibs, blueberries, raspberries, cherries, strawberries, coconut, sprinkles
(yes, they have organic ones)
Use honey instead of maple syrup

Frosting (option 3)
2 tbs. butter - Melt butter in a pan
2 tbs. cocoa
Stir until mixed
Add 1 to 2 cups milk
Stir constantly
Add ¾ cup maple syrup or honey –
'til well blended.
Simmer on low heat 15-40 min.
Stir constantly so it doesn't burn.
Take off when desired consistency is reached.

Variations:
Add chocolate syrup, chocolate chips, cocoa, cacao nibs, blueberries, raspberries, cherries, strawberries, coconut, sprinkles
(yes, they have organic ones)
Use honey instead of maple syrup.

Buckeyes

Ingredients:
1 cup nut butter
½ cup powdered sugar
Chocolate chips melted~

Directions:
Melt chips in a double boiler or very gently over low heat if you don't have one, stirring often.
Once melted, remove from heat.
Blend nut butter and sugar in a bowl until well mixed with your hands is fine (and more fun)
Roll into ½ dollar sized balls
Roll balls in chocolate, this is super messy and KIDS LOVE IT!
Place in freezer 'til set
Roll in powdered sugar

Energy Balls

Ingredients:

1 cup nut butter

1 cup oatmeal

½ cup maple syrup

¼ cup cranberries

¼ cup sliced almonds

½ cup chocolate chips

2 tbs. Chia seeds

Directions:

Blend in a bowl, roll into balls, refrigerate

These have so many possible variations, get creative!

Cheesecake

Ingredients:

2 packages cream cheese

1 8 oz. sour cream

1 cup maple syrup

4 packs graham crackers

1 stick butter

Directions:

Blend graham crackers with melted butter

Press down to form a crust in pie pan

Blend wet ingredients

Pour the cheesecake into pie pan over the crust

Refrigerate 2 hours

Place fruit on top such as kiwi, strawberries, blueberries, oranges, pineapple, etc.

Filling Variations

Chocolate chips, blueberries, strawberries, cherries, cacao nibs

Wildflower Treasure Bites

Preheat oven 350 degrees~

Ingredients:
2 sticks butter or 1 cup coconut oil or 1 cup nut butter
1 cup almond flour
½ cup spelt flour
½ cup all-purpose flour
½ cup coconut flour
¼ cup Flaxseed
1 tbs. Chia seeds
2 tbs. Hempseeds
2 tbs. shredded Coconut
1½ cup maple syrup
2 to 4 tbs. Safflower oil

Almost a whole bag of chocolate chips (doesn't seem like you ever really need that many)
2 tbs. cacao nibs
¼ cranberries
¼ sliced almonds (variations: walnuts, pecans, cashews)

Directions:
Mix all ingredients together
Make little cookie sized patties
Cook for 8 minutes or until golden
They could eat these all day long and it would be so good for them, if you want it sugar-free, you could omit the chocolate chips.

Never Had a Problem Before

In this chapter, we learned a little about the differences between prenatal vitamins and how our baby is worth researching and finding the best one for optimum development. We learned the importance of thinking for ourselves and not following along because everyone always did it that way.

I seriously cannot count the times that I've had people tell me, "Well I've never had any problem with this before," I always like to tell them, "Well you just ran into your first one," like the time we told them we're not giving my grandson the vitamin K shot because his mom had been preparing for this moment for months by drinking Nettle tea so that her blood would clot after birth and so would his. We actually had the nurse tell me he was going to give him the shot after my daughter and son-in-law had just told him no.

And I said, "Ok, then if you give him that shot, can you guarantee me beyond a shadow of a doubt that nothing will happen to him if you give it to him because he already has vitamin K in his body?" And he said, "No," and we told him to go take a hike, he's OUR baby!

So many things that they do at the hospital are just dinging up the insurance with procedures and medications, they have them, they want to use them. That's why if you choose not to have a home birth, look for a birthing center, a place that is not full of sick people around your fresh little piece of heaven.

Question at every turn what and why they are doing everything and if you don't want it, decline. You don't even have to explain, it's your experience, your money. Research and know what you want before you get there with your birth plan in place.

Birth Plan

For instance, if you don't want your baby taken from you as soon as they're born and wish them to be placed on your chest so that the two of you can bond, quietly; then say so. Sure they might be a little bloody, but this is just the beginning of you two sharing lots and lots of body fluid together, so you might as well get used to and hold that little being that you've been carrying around, talking to, singing to, don't let anyone take them away right away unless it's a medical emergency. The first place your baby needs to be is with you.

Then you could both take some Homeopathic Arnica, 4 pellets for you, one for the baby, next some Rescue Remedy. Sit quietly and feel each other's skin, the beating of your hearts together, feeling the separation that exists but is not yet broken. Then they can cut the cord, your body will naturally start pushing out the placenta as the baby latches on.

My poor daughter had her doctor practically rip hers out after I tried telling him, I had 3 daughters and I've been to other births and they never did that! He wouldn't stop. That's why hopefully if you have a Midwife in place, she can advocate for you if you are at the hospital.

What's right for me is not right for every woman, my intention is to create a space in your brain, where you think about your birth and what you want and what you definitely don't want. Certain music? Candles, (if you're at home), salt lamps can be brought into a hospital or birthing center, we have even been at some hospitals that have had salt lamps at the nursing station.

What's important to you? Create that space and make sure that the people supporting you are aware of your intentions and wishes. Make your birth the best memory of your life.

Unfortunately, I have heard stories of women who didn't have any birth plan in place and without it, anything can happen, when you're in labor is not a time for you to be giving directions. It's a time when everything needs to be to your specifications so that you feel as comfortable as possible for the most memorable day of your life.

Remember this is their job, they're there every day, in the end they really don't care, it's your experience, they are merely there to facilitate it and if someone makes you uncomfortable, tell the nurse who doesn't that you don't need the other one's help anymore, someone else will be fine. Don't let anyone undermine your special time, they are at work, they might be having a bad day, that's ok, it's just not your problem. You need to like everyone in the room.

Chapter 2 ~ From the Beginning

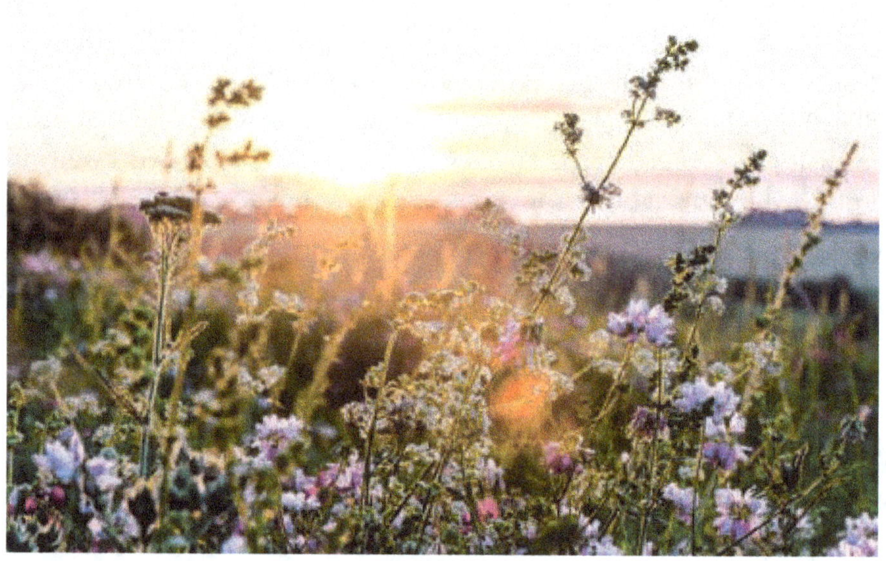

*"Let the children be free; encourage them;
let them run outside when it is raining;
let them remove their shoes when they find a puddle of water;
and when the grass of the meadows is wet with dew,
let them run on it and trample it with their bare feet;
let them rest peacefully when a tree invites them to sleep beneath its shade;
let them shout and laugh when the sun wakes them in the morning."*
                                                                    -Maria Montessori

In this chapter, we will begin to understand how long the relationship between humans and the plant kingdom has lasted and how it has stood the test of time. We will understand the subtle nuances of plants and notice the similarities in perceptions of plants from around the world. A little history of herbs is included along with the background and basis for understanding the world of Holistic Herbal Healing and who the important founders of medicine were.

We'll open ourselves to the herbal translation of Mother Nature's subtle yet obvious system of The Doctrine of Signatures, what Folk Medicine is will be understood, an introduction to the ancient knowledge of Ayurvedic Medicine will be given, a basic understanding of how and when it shifted from natural herbal medicine to chemical medications is laid down as well as the underlying deceit that is the foundation of synthetic, chemical medications and the introduction to their own medical term for 'doctor induced disease'= Iatrogenic Disease…..

History

In the beginning, plants were the only form of medicine and herbal remedies were the medicine that was taught and used. Plants have been used for 60,000 years. The oldest written herbal known is, *The Ebers Papyrus*, written around 1500 BCE, naming more than 125 plants with over 800 prescriptions for poultices, salves, enemas, suppositories, pills, gargles, salves, inhalations, liquid medicines and directions for fumigation.

Epiduras was the first spa, founded in the sixth century BCE in Greece, by Aesculapius, the ancient Greek God of Medicine, son of the God, Apollo and the nymph Coronis, utilizing herbal decoctions, baths, fasting, sea breezes with fresh mountain air, along with the therapeutic use of drama, games and music.

The ruins can still be seen, including a large stone slab with famous cures from over 400 herbs inscribed into it. Thales of Miletus and Pythagoras of Samos compiled these 600 years later. There were many other sanatoriums like the Epiduras throughout Greece who kept meticulous records of disease and treatments. The study of these records gave birth to the art of diagnosing and the study of the natural history of disease.

Known as the Father of Medicine, Hippocrates who coined the lifesaving saying, 'Let food be thy medicine, let thy medicine be thy food,' preserved ancient Greek and Roman medical practices in his teachings.

The Greek physician, Discorides, wrote the first European treatise on the properties and uses of medicinal plants in the first century.

CE, this included more than 500 plants, known as *De Materia Medica*.

He was also the first to write in 65 CE of a cryptic code in Nature he called a signature, 'The Herb Scorpius resembles the tail of the Scorpion, and is good against his biting.' Medieval European physicians named this system, The Doctrine of Signatures, and finetuned the system.

Published in 1290, the Italian physician, Guilielmus of Saliceto wrote a book referring to signature qualities in medicinal plants. The concept was popularized in Europe by Paracelsus in the sixteenth century. But this system was already in use all over the world interpreting resemblances.

Traditional Chinese Medicine interpreting it slightly differently: asserting that plant roots prove useful to treat internal ailments leaving the above-ground flowers, leaves, and seeds better for the treatment of external conditions, such as upper respiratory problems.

Doctrine of Signatures

Divine intervention indicates a subtle yet effective methodology for implicating the best way to locate the chosen plant for a specific ailment or symptom you are trying to treat. Otherwise, if it were not for the sacred act of passing down knowledge through oral traditions, inscribing ancient texts, or deciphering cave drawings, the inherent benefits for each plant might have been lost.

But Mother Nature has designed a simple system to ensure the integrity and sustainability of natural plant medicine throughout the ages even if there were no ancient texts on hand, or a wise woman nearby, through the Doctrine of Signatures.

Through this intricately intuitive, yet simply obvious system of patterns and correspondences, we can begin to speak Mother Earth's language and understand her subtle nuances, the unsuspecting clues hidden in plain sight by the shape of the plant or the color of a flower.

The fact that a walnut resembles a brain and that it helps develop brain function is a common one that some have heard of before and is no coincidence by any means. This is Mother Nature directing Herbalists to the specific remedy for whatever ails you, even if you didn't have anyone else nearby.

By observing your environment, taking notice of what's around you, opening yourself to the silent language spoken before your eyes that remains hidden as a result of a lack of knowledge, you will begin to sense the cure that you are seeking.

Arnica is an excellent remedy for internal bleeding and bruising. It grows on mountainsides, if you fall, she has your back, literally.

Milkweed when cut produces a milky white substance that is useful in increasing the flow of milk in nursing mothers.

Jewel Weed often grows near Poison Ivy and is an excellent remedy for it.

Ginkgo Biloba improves memory and it's good for your brain while the nut of the tree looks like a brain, also.

Saxifraga derived from the Latin saxum (rock) and frangere (to break), a species of plant that can grow out of cracks in rocks, was interpreted as plants that 'break rock', as being helpful in removing kidney stones.

Mushrooms when sliced you will see the resemblance to a human ear, it serves as one of the few foods that contain vitamin D, which has been found to improve hearing and is important for healthy bones, including the tiny ones in your ear that transmit sound to the brain.

Sweet **potatoes** resembling the pancreas, actually balance the glycemic index of diabetics.

Celery, Bok Choy, Rhubarb resembling the fibrous texture of bones, specifically target bone strength. Bone being 23% sodium and celery being 23% sodium is no coincidence. Without enough sodium in your diet, the body pulls it from your bones, resulting in weak, brittle bones.

Avocados take exactly nine months to grow from blossom to ripened fruit and help women shed unwanted birth weight, balance hormones, deter cervical cancer.

Kidney beans improve the health of and maintain optimum kidney function, looking exactly like human kidneys.

Olives are beneficial for women's health and optimum functioning of the ovaries.

Ginger, resembling the stomach, is known for its benefits in aiding digestion, useful for nausea during motion sickness.

Grapes are similar to alveoli, which are tiny bunches of tissues that allow oxygen to pass from the lungs to the bloodstream. Diets high in fresh grapes have been shown to reduce the risk of lung cancer and emphysema. Grape seeds contain proanthocyanidin which appears to reduce the severity of allergy triggered asthma.

Figs hang in twos when they grow, full of seeds that are known to increase the mobility of male sperm increasing numbers of sperm.

Beets are blood red resembling our blood and they are excellent blood builders and blood purifiers.

Eyebright is an herb that resembles an eyeball that is beneficial for the eyes and improves eyesight.

Horsetail is high in silica which is beneficial for the hair.

Carrots, being good for our eyes, when sliced, the core of a carrot resembles an eyeball.

Tomatoes have four distinct chambers just like a human heart, balancing cholesterol, blood pressure, inflammation and reducing the risk of a heart attack.

Ben Charles Harris, in *The Compleat Herbal* (1972), recommends that the first signature one look for is the habitat of an herb:

'Plants that grow in turgid brooks, wet lowlands, and swamps are associated with diseases of wetness: rheumatic disorders, feverish colds, and coughs. These plants include the Willow, Water Pepper, Mints, Verbena, Sweet Flag, Elder, Boneset, Jack-in-the-pulpit, and Skunk Cabbage.

Mucky soil signifies mucous excretions. When mucous excretions are excessive, an inflammation occurs along the membranes of the respiratory and genito-urinary passages which often develop into a diseased condition. The Eucalyptus and Sunflower are often cultivated in swampy areas to rid the places of foul, miasmatic conditions, and are similarly employed to cleanse out the 'swampy' areas of the body.

Herbs and shrubs found growing on the banks of clear ponds and fast-moving brooks are mostly indicated as diuretics, such as Horsetail, Bedstraw, assorted aromatic Mints, Smartweed, Black Alder, Water Agrimony, and Hydrangea. These plants can help to cleanse the urinary system of its waste and stone-forming deposits.

Herbs inhabiting gravelly places may also be found growing over large rock formations or completely covering sandy, barren areas. Such plants can help cleanse and remove from the mucous linings and from their associated areas (i.e., the alimentary and bronchial systems) the harmful stone-forming and catarrhal accumulations. An inflammation may be reduced and disease be prevented by the use of the following: Bearberry, Horsetail, Peppergrass, Parsley, Parsley Piert, Shepherd's Purse, Juniper, May Flower, Gromwell, and the two 'stone-breakers', Sassafras and Saxifrage.'

Folk Medicine

Folk medicine or the household use of herbal remedies was the first medicine and dates back to prehistoric times supporting many settled and traveling herbalists. In the fourth century BCE, Theophrastus wrote the Greek book that founded the science of Botany, *Historia Plantarum*.

We have the ancient monasteries to thank for diligently hand copying manuscripts from historic Greek and Roman texts when the Christian church preferred faith healing over the formal practice of medicine. The monasteries then became a local hub of medical knowledge; their luscious herb gardens provided the herbal remedies for most disorders.

If not the monasteries, folks turned to the 'wise women' of the village seeking their secret remedies of herbal lore passed down for generations including enchantments and spells. These were the 'wise women' who became the targets and victims of the hysteria of the Inquisitions and Witch Trials in the Middle Ages.

For example, if you take St. John's wort flowers and put them in olive oil or any other kind of oil and set that jar in front of a window, the liquid will turn red over a period of time, even though the flowers are yellow. This has nothing to do with Witchcraft, Sorcery or the Devil.

This is a result of the substance found in the plant called Hypericin. Hypericin is known to be a potent antiviral, antidepressant, antimicrobial, etc.

Because of this compound changing the oil from yellow flowers to red meant the loss of many women's lives, it meant that these women were demons, possessed and working for and with the Devil, whom most of them didn't even acknowledge as he is within the Christian religion, which most of them weren't apart of and so they were called 'witches' and were executed. Sadly, many of the 9,000,000 women who were executed during the Witch Trials were Herbalists and women who knew the craft of herbs.

The anonymous *Grete Herball* of 1526 was the first Herbal to be published in English with two more following that are probably the two best known Herbals in English: the first in 1597 by John Gerard titled: *The Herbal or General History Of Plants* and then *The English Physician Enlarged* in 1653 by Nicholas Culpepper.

Enjoying phenomenal popularity despite being ridiculed by the peers of his day, mostly in retaliation for translating their Latin book of official medicines into English, Culpepper's blend of astrology, folklore, magic, and traditional medicine remained a favorite.

An herb in the Middle Ages might be prescribed by a peasant grandmother, sold by a traveling herbalist, charmed to be an ingredient in a magical potion or brew by a 'wise women' or quack, or pulverized into a repulsive and complex blend to be applied by a physician with hopes of bringing relief.

A Story about the Black Death

In the fourteenth century, you might've heard of the Black Death, Black Plague, etc. It was a pandemic that went through Europe and Asia killing A LOT of people. There were four thieves or grave robbers who were stealing from the dead bodies and their homes but weren't getting sick. How did they do it?

When they were caught, they gave up their secret in an effort to save their lives. The Secret was a blend of herbs blended with vinegar. A famous French chemist and scholar, René-Maurice Gattefossé, who is regarded as the Father of Aromatherapy, published the original recipe that was hung in the museum of Old Marseille in France in his book from 1937 Gattefossés Aromatherapy. This is the recipe that was posted in France long ago.

Take three pints of strong white wine vinegar, add a handful of each of wormwood, meadowsweet, wild marjoram and sage, fifty cloves, two ounces of campanula roots, two ounces of angelic, rosemary and horehound and three large measures of camphor. Place the mixture in a container for fifteen days, strain and express then bottle. Use by rubbing it on the hands, ears, and temples from time to time when approaching a plague victim.

Paracelsus

The downfall of herbal medicine began as early as the seventeenth century with the introduction by the physician Paracelsus of utilizing active chemical drugs such as arsenic, copper sulfate, iron, sulfur and mercury as healing substances.

Too bad his other beliefs corresponding to plants didn't stick. He believed that through the wise use of plants, whose properties correspond to their ruling planet, a beneficial astral influence would be directed into the body neutralizing disease.

He taught that there was a vital essence in all living things he called, 'mumia' and that the Universe was a manifestation of this life force which acted through differentiated forms. Believing that food was an important factor contributing to man's health recognizing that spark in all living things, which is the opposite of physicians today, regarding the Universe as an accumulation of forms which can be considered separately and treated without regard for a unifying force.

Ayurvedic Medicine

Ayurvedic medicine is an ancient holistic medical science of life, foundations trace back to the second century BCE. Teachings about the healing properties of the herbs were composed in the form of poems, called 'Shlokas' used by Sages describing the use of medicinal plants.

This Hindu system of healing is based upon four eminent compilations of knowledge (Vedas) known as Yajur Veda, Rig Veda, Sam Veda and Atharva Veda. Rig Veda is the most well-known of all the four Vedas and describes 67 plants and 1,028 Shlokas.

The Atharva Veda and Yajur Veda describe 293 and 81 medicinally useful plants. This system is still in use today with many traditional Ayurvedic herbs and remedies infiltrating the medical systems around the world that are just learning of their practices, beginning to understand what they have known all along.

Homeopathy

In the nineteenth century, Samuel Hanneman founded the system of Homeopathy. Within this system, herbs are prepared in minuscule doses. By the time the process of dilution is complete, there is no more plant matter left in the remedy. It is the 'essence of the plant' that remains. By utilizing these minuscule doses, he achieved great results healing symptoms and disorders.

His method of healing was to give minuscule doses of a plant that would elicit the same effect as the symptom he was trying to treat in a healthy person. By administering it to someone who was experiencing those symptoms, the effect causing the opposite reaction resulted in the diminishment of those symptoms.

Before administration, he would ask them a large number of questions for about an hour, in an effort to identify the person's constitution, such as, "Does it feel better with hot or cold?" "Do you like a blanket or no blanket?" Really specific questions, he would then turn to the Materia Medica which holds the properties of all of the plants along with their specific constitutions.

Being an intensive process, he would match the remedy specific for that person's constitution. He taught that the body has a 'Vital Force' that when stimulated by Homeopathic remedies triggers healing. This model of medicine and philosophy of healing has enjoyed great success for over 200 years.

Vital Force

Herbs stimulate the body's Vital Force. Our 'Vital Force' has been called Chi in China, Prana in India, although not exactly the same, they are similar. All cultures have a name for this life force or energy that stimulates healing in the body.

Many cultures have ancient texts with stories of herbs being used ceremoniously and medicinally for thousands of years to shift the body and the mind into another mode of thinking, being, or perceiving your environment.

By removing blockages, stimulating necessary systems, or suppressing unnecessary hormones, herbs allow us to heal from the inside out without suppressing our body's natural function.

Iatrogenic Disease

Many cancers in America are medically induced from drugs or radiation. Iatrogenic disease is a term used to describe doctor induced illness. Can you believe there is actually a medical 'term' or 'diagnosis' for what we should basically be calling malpractice?

Only 42-46% of cancer patients die from Cachexia, which is from actual cancer which would be from losing all of their lean body mass. This means that what kills the majority of cancer patients is pneumonia, liver failure, kidney failure, sepsis, etc. which are mostly all associated with chemotherapy and radiation treatment.

After 5 years of chemo, there's only a 2.1% survival rate. In a study done by Epidemiologists who themselves were doctors, they found that 90% of people who underwent chemotherapy treatments died within 5 years of treatment. This study was published in the 2004 edition of the Journal of Oncology. Damaging DNA, chemo and radiation have a very high propensity to create secondary cancers.

Which is why they do not say you are cured until you are 5 years out, otherwise, they call it remission, fully expecting it to come back. A good indication of the toxicity is the fact that they have to suit up to administer it to you.

But what happened, anyway? Why is it that 1 in 4 people will get cancer, these statistics are very different than they were 100 years ago? For starters, our grandparents grew most of their food, there were not all of the refined food choices that we have now, there were not all of the chemical pesticides and fertilizers that there are now. The destruction of our food supply began over 50 years ago.

Summary ~

In this chapter, we explored the periods of time and influential figures in the world of herbs, as well as the origins of many of our new healing modalities. The thousands of plants that have been recorded over time by a number of Herbalists and Scholars would not have made it into our pharmacopeia had it not been for them.

We have them to thank for had it not been for them taking the time to record their results from each plant over a millennium, much of that ancient knowledge would have been lost.

But we now know thanks to Mother Nature's hidden, yet visible subliminal dialect of signatures known as the Doctrine of Signatures that all we really need to achieve healing with our remedies as Herbalists, is to observe her in her entirety never leaving anything to chance or assuming, as her language is so literal that even a child could understand it.

Chapter 3 ~ The Downfall of Our Food Supply

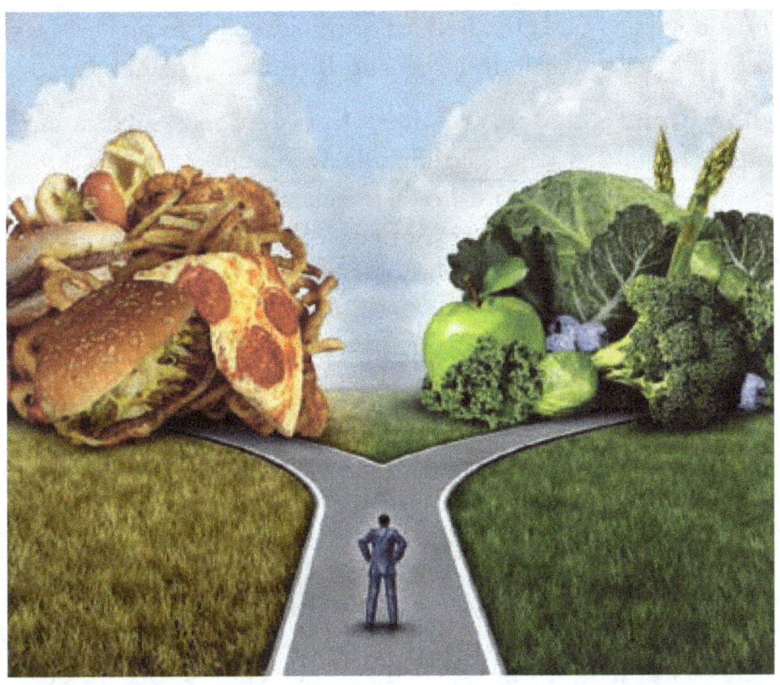

"There is a growing body of evidence that ultra-processed foods are deliberately designed to be addictive – similar to cigarettes and alcohol – and are major contributors to the twin epidemics of obesity and diabetes in our country."

— *Sen. Bernie Sanders*

In this chapter, we will explore the downfall of our countries food supply and understand its shady beginnings and motivations with an understanding that our health is not at the forefront of what is being considered when it comes to the production of our food.

A foundation will be laid grasping the motivation behind it all and knowing the sad truth that America is one of the few countries that allow this level of contamination and poison in their food, not only disregarding American's health but profiting from the diseases that their poisons cause.

We begin to understand why the emphasis on organic is so crucial after being introduced to GMOs, chemical pesticides and fertilizers as well as the destruction of the meat industry and then the dairy industry.

We'll know by the end of this chapter why if we don't make sure that we are eating organic that we could literally be serving human waste at our dinner table. And how easy it is to just pack a lunch or go out of our way to make sure what we're eating is not tainted and how we have the ability to change our gene expression through Epigenetics and that NO ONE is bound by 'bad genes'.

America's Health

Why is it that so many Americans are so sick? With all of the new technologies now, you would think that people are living longer, but they're not. Along with the steady decline of our food we have seen the steady decline of our health as a nation. Is this just a coincidence? Seeing as how I don't believe in coincidences; I believe it rather obviously not. Coincidence could mean it was by chance.

The decline of a nation's health is no coincidence or even a quandary. We know why, there are many contributing factors, lack of exercise, environmental factors, lifestyle choices, food, dehydration, emotions, etc. Many of the diseases that plague Americans today are a direct result of choices that they are making every day.

Why do I limit this to mostly Americans, you ask? Probably because many other countries do not allow these toxic food additives that we not only allow, but we bank on. Not only do we allow these cheap artificial fillers in our food increasing shareholders' pockets, but then we bank on the inherent sicknesses they cause and diseases they contribute to.

Cancer is the second largest industry in America next to petrochemicals. Guess what's in just about any personal care product that you pick up in any grocery store? Petrochemicals, you see they get you coming and going.

Not Allowed-Some other countries do not allow these kinds of poisons, such as GMOs in their country and a long list of other carcinogenic ingredients that we allow, into their food supply and personal care products.

Funding for their citizen's healthcare, it is not in their interest to poison their citizens. Nestle, Hershey's and many other huge food conglomerates produce different food that they ship overseas. They give us the poison and ship the non-tainted food across the ocean to other countries that actually care about their country's health as a nation.

WHY?

If people actually believed that if they ate better, they would feel better, would they really be on so many prescriptions? Why wouldn't they just change their diets if that's the case? Because it has been sent in a subliminal message that you have NO control over your body and what sickness or diseases you get.

Not that the majority of contributing diseases that result in a loss of life could have been prevented. No one wants to hear that. It's much easier to feel like you were blindsided with poor health, like you never saw it coming.

But research now shows us that we can't hide our heads in the sand and say we didn't know. Why do you think McDonald's is selling organic coffee? Because they care? No, because they know that the new generation is going to be healthier, is going to be more educated. Look you are reading this book right now, educating yourself so that you will be healthier and with this knowledge you will affect change.

Remember that the majority of deficiencies are not caused by a specific nutrient missing from our diet; it is the direct result of a breakdown of the physical metabolism. And that with an adequate diet our bodies have the capacity to manufacture the proper vitamins required to maintain optimal health.

Our bodies give us signals; disease is a message. It begins a much needed journey. It means it's time for a change - of either pace or scenery. Pain is our friend; it's a warning, listen to it. It serves a purpose, it's our bodies' lingo for telling us we are either overdoing it and need to slow down or that we are not doing enough whether it's exercise, eating, sleeping, etc. When we eat certain foods that make us feel bad or that cause inflammation and after we eat, we wonder why we don't feel good, we can't pretend we don't know why.

It is very unfortunate that our food supply is so tainted. If you do not know what I am referring to, read on.

Nutrition

Around the turn of the century, when they started devitalizing flour and rice, folks actually got Beriberi because their bodies were so lacking in nutrients. So, what did they do once they put 2 and 2 together? Stop bleaching it? No! They just 'fortified' it! The US public health service in 1919 announced a definite connection between over refined flour and the diseases of Beriberi and Pellagra both vitamin deficiency diseases of which over 100,000 cases were reported in Mississippi alone.

Developing enriched white bread, instead of just refraining from bleaching it leaves you with nothing but raw starch, which has so little nutrient value that bacteria won't even eat it. Adding vitamins back in, which are synthetic in origin, is not the same as the nutritive values found naturally in the plant. Silos containing this enriched grain remain undisturbed by rodents.

A wheat berry contains all of the essential enzymes, vitamins and minerals such as copper, iron, cobalt, manganese and molybdenum in the germ and husk. Ever wonder why bread was referred to as, 'the staff of life?' Wheat germ contains the entire vitamin B complex and is one of the very few places where it is found in Nature.

Not to mention it contains barium which is a mineral found in whole wheat and a deficiency in this can result in cardiac disease. Instead of just leaving the rice unpolished or the wheat germ and bran intact, they enriched the bleached, devitalized product so that now it did have the same vitamins that they took out. But as I keep repeating, our bodies do not know how to utilize these synthetic compounds.

Hydrogenated Fats

Hydrogenated fats consisting of using heated nickel catalyst to force hydrogen into the gaps between the carbon atoms of linoleic acid, hydrogen destroys essential fatty acids. Because it is non-absorbable by the body's cells, it ends up lining the blood vessels leading to heart disease.

Perhaps being the foremost precursor in heart disease if for no other reason than it is contained within everything in a general grocery store including shortening, commercial bakery products, peanut butter, bread, cookies, crackers, snack foods, most drinks, etc.

Rice

Rice is one of the best foods in the World, one of the richest sources of natural vitamin B complex, rice has been bleached to nothing more than rice starch devoid of any vitamins or nutritious value. In the Philippines, American missionary wives managed to kill off hundreds of prisoners in the local jails by basically substituting polished rice for natural rice in the prisoner's diet thus causing Beriberi.

Peanut Butter

Mostly being made from rancid peanuts since we have learned to clean it up, deodorize it and color it so that it can be sold to unsuspecting mothers, adding hundreds of toxic additives. This makes it nearly impossible for the citizen to tell that the food is going or has already gone bad. Conventional (not organic) peanuts are known to contain large quantities of chemical pesticides and should be avoided.

Devitalized Carbohydrates

One downfall in the destruction of our food included bleaching sugar, removing the molasses, vitamins and minerals leaving only carbohydrates and calories. Allowing it to keep better, it can be stored for years.

White sugar contributes to the depletion of vitamins and minerals. One can of Coke contains enough sugar to break down half of your immune system for four hours. Immunosuppressed or immuno- compromised patients cannot afford to have this lapse. And that is just the sugar of one Coke, not including all the artificial sweeteners or other sugars that other foods are laden with that might be included in the diet.

Artificial sweeteners unlike natural fruit sugars, maple syrup, molasses and honey, go straight into the bloodstream causing instant hyperglycemia or too much sugar in the blood, drowning the human cells in sugar. Heeding the alarm, the pancreas puts out too much insulin and produces a state of hypoglycemia or too little sugar in the blood.

In the 1940s, we started seeing the sharply increased dietary intake of refined, devitalized carbohydrates. Devitalized carbohydrates interfere with total body immunity by contributing to the destruction of white blood cells, depleting minerals and vitamins, weakening of body tissues; ligaments, skin, muscle, collagen, etc.

These refined, toxic substances masquerading as foods include but are not limited to white sugar (glucose, maltose, fructose, corn syrup, corn sweeteners, high fructose corn syrup, dextrose, high maltose corn syrup, maltodextrin, sorbitol, maltitol, erythritol, glucitol, maltitol, xylitol, lactitol), artificial sweeteners such as:

- Acesulfame Potassium - Sunnett, Sweet One,

- Aspartame - Nutrasweet, Equal,

- Neotame - N/A,

- Saccharin - Sweet 'N Low, Sweet Twin, Sugar Twin,

- Sucralose - Splenda and white flour, non-whole-grain pasta, white rice, most vegetable oils, including hydrogenated and trans fats, refined salt and others.

Iodized Salt

Some know that table salt is not good for you and others think the small amount of salt that they use, could not possibly be significant, but over time, it can cause high blood pressure and heart disease.

Containing trace minerals in balance, sea salt is very good for you, but by the time it's been refined and reaches the table, it's nothing more than sodium chloride devoid of minerals. Then it is treated with a drying agent under high heat to make it free flowing, actually disturbing the delicate balance of sodium and potassium in the cells of the heart.

(GMOs) Genetically Modified or Engineered Organisms

Devitalized carbohydrates were just the beginning of a new era of toxic, cancer causing culprits in the downfall of our health as a nation. When the first EKG was brought to the states, there was no heart disease to be monitored; now heart disease is one of the leading causes of death in the US.

In less than 100 years, that is a pretty devastating statistic, if you really think about it! Now it would seem that devitalized carbohydrates are the least of our worries with GMOs (genetically modified or engineered organisms) arriving on the scene.

What does this mean? It means that in a lab they are genetically modifying our food. An example of this would be taking a gene from the 'Flounder' fish and inserting it into a tomato so that the tomato can withstand frigid weather. Most of the corn, soy, wheat and sugar beets, which are what a lot of white sugar is derived from, are genetically modified. Not with fish genes or anything, though.

They are genetically modifying it so that it can withstand a horrific, cancer causing pesticide known as Round-Up or glyphosate made by Monsanto (who was recently bought by Bayer). Round-Up causes a bug's stomach to explode. By spraying this on the crops, it kills the bugs but not the plants because they are supposed to be resistant to it.

So, these plants that are genetically modified to be glyphosate resistant, turns out really aren't food at all. Food by definition means a substance that sustains life. This 'food' not only does not sustain life, but actually destructs life. It is destructive to life, to human tissue, it causes inflammation, leaky gut, digestion issues, joint pain, headaches, allergies, etc.

Remember that inflammation is the root of all disease, so if what we are eating is causing inflammation, then what we are eating is causing disease in our body. Food can either be the most potent form of medicine or it can be the slowest form of poison.

Plants absorb whatever medium they are grown in. Have you ever seen carnations colored pink, blue, green and wonder how they do that? Different varieties? No, but good guess, they put food coloring in the water and the flower absorbs it. So, we know that these plants are absorbing the glyphosate. There's actually research now proving that landscapers and other folks who work with Round-Up have a higher chance of getting lymphoma from the Round-Up.

But this is really just the tip of the iceberg. We can see the ripple effect reaching our pollinators, birds and wild animals eat the corn grown in fields, not only deer, but turkeys, moose, bears, all of the animals that people hunt. So, for people who are trying to be conscious and not eat meat from the grocery store and go shoot their own food – they've ruined that wild game as well. Today, if you eat wild animals living where corn is grown nearby, you are eating Round-Up.

And when it rains, the runoff goes into our brooks and waterways, polluting the fish and other sea creatures. We are all connected in an intricate web of life that all depend on each other. Not to mention the pollen from those GMO fields blowing in the wind and pollinating organic farmers' fields who don't want any part of that poison on their fields.

Monsanto has gone so far as to sue a farmer for growing their corn, because of cross pollination in a counter lawsuit from an organic farmer who tried to sue them for ruining his organic crop.

Not only is the soil drenched with chemicals, but the plants grown in them are loaded with the chemical as well. The deterioration of our soil leads to food that is void of vitamins and minerals. Food that has been tested over time with decades apart has shown a steady decline of nutrients in our food supply.

Here's an excellent resource for learning more about the health risks associated with GMOs, follow this link to watch Genetic Roulette, The Gamble Of Our Lives with Jeffrey Smith.

https://www.youtube.com/watch?v=7sUNxX0OxP8

Organic

But not all plants are the same. By choosing organic food, we are making a conscious choice to eat unadulterated food grown in its purest form without the use of carcinogenic pathogens that hide in plain sight, under a cloak labeled pesticides and fertilizers.

For example, they say carrots are high in vitamin A, right? Oranges are high in vitamin C, but if these plants were grown under toxic conditions in depleted vitamin void soil, then how much vitamin A or vitamin C is the plant really going to contain? Compare this to a plant that is grown in vital soil full of the necessary components to guarantee plant nutrition, and that is balanced by all of the microorganisms in the soil feeding off of each other.

If for some reason organic is out of reach, like it was for us when we were living in Missouri for 2 months, with NO organic food anywhere in sight, non-GMO is the next best option. Look for the butterfly in a little box with the letters non-GMO quality assurance label.

I've heard people say that they don't believe organic is really any different, believe me, it is! As an organic producer, my records are scrutinized every year with traceability audits, record checking, lab inspection, product inspection, label approval, there's ALOT that goes into it. I assure you, it is very different from produce that is not organic.

Meat Industry

Briefly, I'd like to discuss the whole meat/chicken industry. Protein is one of the most important items in the human diet providing eight essential amino acids, the building blocks of the body. There are twenty-two amino acids. Eight are called essential for the adult, ten are necessary for growing children. With these, the body can build the others.

The most popular form of protein in the United States is beef that has been force-fed for 180 days with low quality protein hybrid grains sprayed with poisonous insecticides that go straight into the fat of the meat specifically into the marbling leading straight to heart disease.

In an effort to add extra weight on cattle and produce a multi-million dollar profit, cattle raisers fed their animals DES or diethylstilbestrol which can be carcinogenic in both men and women.

Finally banned in the spring of 1973, it was replaced by a compound called Sinovec, which contains estradiol benzoate. This compound is considered by many experts to be cancer causing. Not to mention the sixteen other drugs singly or in combination which the FDA suspects are carcinogenic when ingested by humans that are being ingested by beef steers, hogs, sheep and poultry.

Organ meat should only be eaten if the animal was fed organically. Livers, being the main filters, contain the majority of toxins that the animal was exposed to. Commercially grown chickens have arsenic and stilbestrol in their bodies much of which winds up in the liver.

Chickens are kept in tiny little boxes so that they can fatten up quickly given large quantities of growth hormones, not even having enough room to raise their wings. If that was the quality of life of the animals you are eating, then how good do you think it can be for you?

Studies show that the more animal food consumed in a society, the more cancer that is seen in that society. Too much protein elevates blood cholesterol levels. These studies are based on meat that hasn't even been tainted. It is estimated that by the time a meat-eating man reaches the age of forty, he will have 5 lbs. of undigested meat in his system. Knowing the seediness of the industry, it becomes blatantly clear that if you are not eating organic meat, you are creating disease in your body. If you are a big meat eater, or you don't feel like refraining from animal protein, do yourself a favor and buy organic meat and limit your consumption.

Obesity is linked to more than sixty common diseases: two-thirds of adults and one-third of children struggle with obesity. Do you think it could have anything to do with all of the growth hormones? Another coincidence, right?

We now know the toxins found in meat range from antibiotics, to growth hormones but that's not even the worst of it, after an animal dies, instead of just giving it a proper burial, they grind it up and make animal feed out of it. Now if you haven't heard of this, it might be hard for you to believe, it does sound like it's out of a horror movie or a Sci-Fi movie but it is entirely true. If you look up rendering plants, you will see exactly what I am talking about.

Rendering Plants

Rendering plants are where some of the euthanized pets end up, the road-kill, when animals die on farms, those are sent to the rendering plants as well. All of those dead, diseased, sick animals are then ground up into feed and fed to animals that eat meat like chicken feed, pig feed, etc. but then it is given to vegetarian animals that should not even be eating meat, such as cows, lambs, sheep. All animal feed has this in it, you can't get away from it.

This partly explains Mad Cow and Mad Sheep disease. There is so much more information about this and how it changes the body's proteins and how toxic these proteins become. These animals are not meant to process animal proteins. There's a lot more to it, but for the scope of this book, that's as deep as we will go and you can research it on your own.

By now, I'd imagine you are starting to see a pattern, a pattern whose tapestry spreads thin, but is a veil and if you don't observe very closely noting each fiber, the minutest of details, adjusting your eyes to the darkness, you might not be able to see it, or worse you won't want to believe it. It's easier to just turn away, pretend you didn't hear it, act like you didn't read it, assuming that it's all going to be okay; but then you start looking around you. You start noticing that everyone you know is either taking a pharmaceutical medication or is complaining about their health.

Could it be the food? Maybe the old saying, 'You are what you eat' holds some weight? Our grandparents and great-grandparents didn't grow up with everyone sick around them. Half of the diseases today weren't even around 100 years ago.

Could it be the fact that everything you're eating is grown in chemical, carcinogenic, cancer causing soil fertilized with cancer causing chemicals and then sprayed with cancer causing pesticides? That is not a rhetorical question.

RBST/RBGH Recombinant Bovine Somatotropin

It's not just the meat industry that they've infiltrated, dairy didn't have a chance either. RBST/RBGH is a hormone given to cows to increase their milk production - approved in 1993 by the FDA.

Cows treated with this hormone began developing many significant health issues with a 50% increase in the risk of lameness (leg and hoof problems), seeing over a 25% increase in the frequency of udder infections (mastitis), and severe animal reproductive problems, such as infertility, cystic ovaries, fetal loss and birth defects. But do you think the FDA pulled it? Or even made mandatory labeling? No.

I remember when this happened in Vermont. We pushed so hard for labeling that I remember walking down the aisle in the store and any dairy product containing this growth hormone had a little blue dot by its price tag. The ENTIRE dairy aisle had one on it! Except for Cabot and Butterworks, they were the only companies that didn't have that blue dot. Well, let me tell you, that didn't last long! That went away and then it took years to get the labeling on each product.

BioSludge

Ok, do you want to hear perhaps the worst degradation of our food supply? Have you ever heard of BioSludge? So, sewage is human waste, right? Well, someone got the idea to take human waste and use it for fertilizer. Mmm, hmmm, that's right, sewage made into fertilizer. Now, personally, I do not like to use manure from animals because I cannot guarantee that they were fed organically, so taking human waste and putting that on my garden would be absolutely absurd.

Animals are way cleaner than people and I wouldn't want that waste on my garden if it's not organic. People use chemicals on their bodies, in their food, even ingest them in their medications. The wrongness of this practice cannot even begin to be touched upon in the scope of this book.

The reasons why this practice is so unheard of could fill a library, but not even just that, what do you feel instinctively when you think of that? Sure, I know that some people have composting toilets and put that on their garden, but usually these people are semi-conscious and that is why they are composting so odds are they are cleaner and it is their waste going on their garden.

For someone who doesn't even like to use animal manure that is not organic on her garden, the idea of using human sewage sludge is just downright repulsive! And when they started this, going around to farms in the Midwest and offering some 'free fertilizer' to farmers, the farmers' families started experiencing unexplained health issues.

When their soil was tested, according to Mike Adams, a scientific researcher specializing in forensic food analysis, there was Benadryl in it, among other toxic substances that you wouldn't water your plants with… much less grow your food in… much less… EAT!

Are you starting to see why I cannot stress the importance of organic, enough, for your family? Before we switched over to completely organic, I remember saying to someone, "Yes, we eat organic food, but not everything. Things that we eat a lot of, we don't eat organic. We eat organic spaghetti sauce, but we don't eat organic butter. We eat way too much butter to buy that organic."

No sooner did the words leave my mouth, than I asked myself if I heard what I just said? If you eat that much of it, then that's definitely something your family should be eating organic, right?

My husband tried to tell me at one point that my daughters and I could eat the organic food but he wouldn't, he'd just eat pesticide, chemical fertilizer laden food. At the time, he was the breadwinner of the family, as I homeschooled our daughters. I asked him how that would make any sense?

He was the one keeping the whole family going, supporting us, clearing the snow, cutting wood, working on the cars...we needed him to be healthy out of anyone! He was the backbone of our family. He was just as important as we were! When I put it like that, he understood my position.

Microwave Radiation

In 1967, microwaves were introduced as a 'quick' way to make a meal, no more waiting for your food to heat up. Little did anyone know that eating food that has been microwaved actually changes your blood cells in such a way that can be observed under a microscope.

In other words, if you took a blood sample and looked at your blood under a microscope, your blood cells would look very round and beautifully symmetrical repelling each other with their electrical charge. When you take another blood sample after eating microwaved food, now your blood cells do not look beautiful and perfect. They look all distorted.

This is research that has been around since I received my Homeopathy Certificate and this was a study from another country. Now, there are lots of articles written in the U.S. as to the hazards of these life destructing machines but no one declares a war on them knowing that they are actually destroying human health.

When my daughters were young there was a little girl in our community who got a brain tumor when she was 6 years old. We didn't really know the family, but as community members, we were aware of the little girl. I wondered what conditions in her environment could contribute to the tumor. She lived near where we lived, so I knew there was no toxic water or air contributing to it.

She beat the cancer and grew up and went to high school with my daughters. One day when my daughter was at this girl's house, they were talking about her previous brain tumor. Her father said he swore it had something to do with her standing with her nose at the microwave when they used it. I would have to agree with him.

Better Choices for a New Generation

In the recent past, since the Industrial Revolution and forward, medicine has moved away from the natural world and into the synthetic, chemical world. Long ago, people spent time outdoors, enjoying fresh air, growing their food, life was pretty basic. Once the chemical revolution of synthetic single molecule compounds became the norm, in a way, it removed one's own power to heal themselves.

Before when herbal or folk medicine was the preferred choice, people took responsibility for collecting their herbs, preparing their remedies, eliminating what was necessary, resting and feeling better. It seems like the older generation gave their power over to their 'prescriptions.'

Being told to "take this pill and call me in the morning" has shifted the awareness from preparing your own medicine to trusting someone else with your health and wellness and really expecting to not have to make dietary or lifestyle changes at all.

By taking a 'magic pill,' this 'magic pill' will halt any discomfort we are experiencing and it will do it instantly. Instant gratification is the expectation, now. No more remembering to take your tea or herbal preparation 2 to 3 times a day and feeling the effects over a few days with symptomatic changes slowly decreasing until total health is restored. when they used it. I would have to agree with him.

Small Print

BUT...did you read the small print? Is the relief of removing that symptom worth liver or kidney damage, suicidal thoughts, shortness of breath, swelling over your face, difficulty breathing, lymphoma, brain bleeding, joint pain, insomnia, lethargy, tightness in your chest, restlessness, diarrhea, nervousness, dizziness, stroke, rashes, death even?

Just because you're sad or because you have frequent urination? And it has become so status quo, that these folks who take their prescriptions and follow blindly, completely disregard the side effects and when they do start experiencing them, they don't notice them as being side effects.

They don't understand why they don't feel good, why they don't have energy, why their bones hurt or their joints ache, why they have digestive issues, so they go back to the doctor with new symptoms and the doctor prescribes a new medication to cover those symptoms.

All the while, the person is literally a walking side effect with all of their symptoms stemming from their prescriptions that they've been told that they have to take for the rest of their life.

It is a sad vicious circle, that I have seen all too often with older people. But it doesn't have to be that way, there are as many people who are eighty years old that are not on prescriptions, who get around, travel, exercise and enjoy a great quality of life as those who don't.

By removing these chemicals from our consumption, we can give our livers a chance to process the everyday chemicals produced by the metabolism of the body. Introducing toxins such as prescription medications and chemicals and pesticides in our food, applying them to our skin, breathing them in the air, engaging with toxic people in toxic relationships building stress hormones, all add up at the end of the day to liver toxicity and toxic overload.

As a new generation, we can take our health into our hands and if we start noticing symptoms, maybe we can take an objective look at our life - are we eating right? Drinking enough water? Dehydration can wreak havoc on your body. Sleeping enough? Exercising enough? Meditating?

What is wrong? Figure out what part of your body it is and start taking some supplements whether in a capsule or blend some tea, go buy a tincture, do whatever you have to. Find what you need and give yourself time. Healing is a process, it does not happen overnight.

If, after a short while, you don't notice a difference and you're feeling that bad, sure maybe go see your Healthcare Provider, see what they say after some non-invasive tests. Then re-evaluate; keep up on the same regimen, add another herbal remedy, increase dosage or potency. Know that your body wants to heal and if you give it what it needs, then you will be rewarded with vibrant health.

If you don't listen to your body and you don't give it what it needs, you can be like one of those people with low energy and lots of side effects. The choice is yours, so why not just give yourself a chance? We were not put here to be sick. If we are sick, it is a direct result of our choices.

Take some responsibility for yourself and make the necessary changes to improve not just your diet and your health, but your life and not just your life, but your family's as well. And by making these positive choices, they will not only affect you and your family but the health and well-being of the whole planet. Every decision we make affects the whole whether we choose to acknowledge it or not.

Pack a Lunch

You can read about it, you can watch it, you can listen to family talk about it, but only you will be the one when you're hungry next time and you're out, who will be the one who makes a responsible choice for the betterment of your family's health. If you just reach for the first thing available, it will almost always be something laden with GMOs, high fructose corn syrup and growth hormones.

Or will you go OUT of your way, if necessary, to find the nearest health food store or Natural Food Coop, or VEGAN Cafe to grab lunch? Will you go into the closest grocery store, into the 'organic' aisle and buy some organic fruit and snacks or better yet, pack some organic food with you when you go out, so you know when they're hungry, you are not at the mercy of what conglomerate is closest to you.

When my girls were little and when my husband had cancer, I always packed food and water with us, so that if they were hungry, I knew I wasn't going to offer them poison as a last resort because of my lack of preparation. Living remotely, with the nearest health food store forty-five minutes away, healthy food was not an option generally when we were out.

Age of Information

This is a new decade, not even just a new year; we can bring it in with a new perspective on health, a new outlook of being aware that our health is the result of our choices. A new accountability for our actions, a new responsibility to the planet as a whole.

A new understanding that every choice we make every day has an impact. That it doesn't matter what we've done, it matters what we do now. We know that it is our choices that decide how our genes express themselves.

Epigenetics

Epigenetics is the science of gene expression. No one is condemned to poor health because of their genes. Epigenetics proves to us that through nutrients, intention and thoughtful dedicated action we can change our gene expression. This means that we are not bound by the choices our ancestors made, we are forging our own path, for our own health, for our own destiny. Nothing is predestined by the faults of our ancestors.

Summary ~

In this chapter, we learned about the decline of our food supply, how we strayed from growing food to processing food. How we slowly moved farther and farther away from raw, natural food in an unadulterated state. The way chemicals have infiltrated not just our soil but our food, every aspect of it.

We learned of the destruction of the wheat berry and the process of bleaching our food. We learned how hydrogenated fats are not readily absorbed by the body lining the blood vessels contributing to heart disease. We learned how they've sprayed peanuts so bad that now even peanut butter isn't good for you if it's not organic.

We've explored how devitalized carbs are hidden by many names but the fact remains that they undermine immunity, destructing white blood cells, weakening the body's tissues, ligaments, etc., deplete vitamins and minerals. We have a basic understanding of how artificial sweeteners differ from natural sweeteners going straight into the bloodstream causing instant hyperglycemia or too much sugar in the blood, drowning the human cells in sugar.

We know that the little bit of table salt that we use is devoid of any trace minerals and adds up over time. We are now aware of glutamate and the role it plays in contributing to the growth of cancer.

We are now aware of glyphosate, Monsanto, Round-Up, GMOs and the disease they can cause in our bodies.

Familiarizing ourselves with the abuse animals in the industry are subjected to between tight quarters and growth hormones to eating the ground up flesh of other animals that are packed into pellets and called goat and other feed.

We've been introduced to the horrors of not only chemical farming but to farming with human feces and now understand why lettuce, tomatoes, spinach, etc. crops end up with E. coli in them. E. coli is feces. How do the vegetables end up with this?? Biosludge! Make sure you wash your veggies REALLY good if they're not organic! Yuck!

We learned how our country has turned its back on keeping our foods and personal care products safe. Hopefully, you now have an understanding of what organic means.

How microwaves actually change our blood cells on a molecular level. We know the importance of listening to our bodies and why following the signs so that we don't get lost could cost us our lives if we don't and the role Epigenetics plays in our gene expression.

Now let's learn about the plants and ways that we can use them to ease our little one's symptoms…

Chapter 4 ~ Preparing Your Remedies

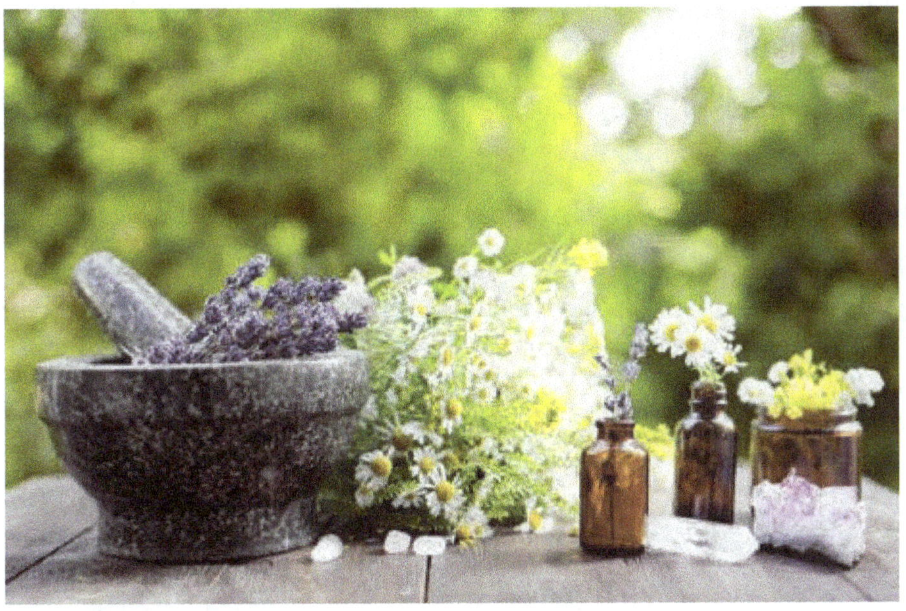

"The art of healing comes from nature, not from the physician. Therefore the physician must start from nature with an open mind."

— *Paracelsus*

In this chapter, we will explore various methods employed in the timeless art of extraction and ways to ensure that you retain as many of the valuable healing properties that herbs possess. We will understand that there is not one way to extract plant compounds, just as important as it is in learning preferences, this education is required in understanding specific methods for each different plant part, as the delicate extraction process of flowers' properties differs from roots and barks.

Introducing the idea that what you're thinking at the time of preparation can increase the efficacy of your remedy. We will learn about Structured Water, what it is, why you should drink it and how easy it is to make. A basic understanding of what the Simpler's Method of Measurements is will also be understood.

One of the best past times as an Herbalist is planning which plant oils you will blend in your next formulation and what it will relieve. There are so many different possible combinations. Herbs, assisting in controlling the course of an illness can give the body the time it needs to restore balance.

The Wonders of Nature

One of the wonders of Nature is the diversity including the various parts of a plant that can be used depending on the specific plant and then the various ways to extract them.

Harvesting

I prefer to harvest according to BioDynamic rhythms; as the moon travels through the sky and crosses into and through the various constellations. If attention is paid as to its placement when planting, harvesting and drying herbs, then the optimum potential of the plant can be reached.

When harvesting garden plants, care should be taken as to which are the strongest if being used for medicine. These will be the first choice. Do not choose plants whose leaves are wilted or that do not look vibrant and healthy.

If harvesting seed, same idea; the best seeds will be from strong, healthy, stocky plants that are flourishing and prolific. Scrawny, mildewed, yellowing, unhealthy plants that are suffering from lack of light or inadequate nutrients or display signs of infestation or any other signs of disease would definitely not be ideal medicine.

Pay attention, taking notice, making mental notes while harvesting, such as thoughts on if next year's herbs might enjoy a different location in the garden or if you need to cut a bush back to supply more light, you can make notes in your garden journal for future adjustments.

Wildcraft

Always begin with native plants in your area. By utilizing local plants that were grown in similar conditions to where you live, these will contain compounds that your body can utilize to boost your immune system. This is much the same as how using local honey decreases the likelihood of allergies developing.

If you notice the native plants in your area, you might not have to take up precious garden space; you can just wildcraft the local herbs around you. Wild herbs are always the best choice for herbal medicines. Although this isn't always possible depending on the season or locale where you are looking.

As a rule, wild plants have more and sometimes even rare curative properties compared to their cultivated counterparts, such as Dandelion, which loses some rare medicinal values that it possesses when grown in the wild in its natural growing environment.

If wildcrafting, take note as to which locations have the healthiest sites and when it is the optimum harvest time. I always thank the plant when harvesting and never take the whole patch. Always leave at least half to grow back for next year. Remember wildcrafting is not isolated to plants; bark and mushrooms, lichen and moss can also be powerful medicine.

Harvesting while observing cosmic rhythms ensures the quality of your herbs due to the unseen astrological influences at play. Plants harvested this way last longer and retain their color longer than others that weren't. Consider other factors when harvesting such as powerlines, traffic, road proximity, neighbors (nuclear power plant.)

Herbs growing in a field will be purer than the ones growing next to the road which is maintained with salt in the winter and herbicides and pesticides for the grass in the summer. The importance of purity in your formulations cannot be stressed enough.

If you are purchasing herbs, under what conditions were they grown? Near or in a city? Or out in the country where there is hopefully no smog, fewer emissions, purer water quality, cleaner air, etc. These are questions you want answered.

Drying

Drying herbs can either be done by air drying, in a dehydrator or with heat. If needed immediately, the herb can be placed in a 200° oven for 20 minutes or until dry. Although this isn't ideal, it can work.

For air drying, herbs should be hung upside down in small, loose bunches in an environment with minimal lights and minimal dust exposure or they can be dried laid out on a screen with plenty of room around each plant. If screens are being utilized, turn herbs every day. Keep flowers and leaves out of Sunlight.

Storing

Dried herbs can be stored, ideally in a paper bag or glass jar, plastic bags can be used but care should be used ensuring that they are BPA-free. Don't want to defeat your purpose by choosing organic seed, using organic amendments on organic soil and then storing it in plastic which has known carcinogens or cancer-causing chemicals present.

Dried herbs can be stored in a cool, dark place or in the freezer. This is my ideal choice to ensure freshness. As stated, paper bags are another option. There are even paper bags with roll tops that have a little window in the front so you can see your herbs, some have a BPA-free lining inside.

Glass jars are also another option, but care needs to be taken that herbs are dried as thoroughly as possible; condensation can result in molding of your medicine.

Herbs should never be kept or stored or prepared near or in a microwave. As medicine, they should never be stored near electrical devices or cell phones, Wi-Fi routers, etc.

Extraction

Extraction is the art of drawing the healing compounds found in plants into a carrier such as oil, alcohol, water or vegetable glycerin. Some herbs are eaten or prepared similarly to food in the same fashion. But when preparing herbs for the very sick or debilitated, extraction is the preferred route.

By removing the fiber and releasing only the beneficial components found in the plant, bypassing all of the waste, direct application of those fortifying compounds can be achieved without the effort of digestion which can steal the bodies energy away from healing during critical moments when the location of the available energy the body has is crucial, allowing it to direct itself into healing as opposed to the fires of digestion.

Because of the multitude of compounds found in herbs and the volatile oil contents, the method of extraction can be critical to the viability of your medicine. If through the extraction process, you are eliminating all or any of the potent benefits, then you are defeating your purpose.

Some herbs should never be simmered and others really require that gentle heat to release those extraordinary compounds. This is where your personal research comes in.

Extraction Methods

Because herbs have so many uses, there are many ways to prepare them for extraction:

- Tincture
- Tea
- Simple
- Decoction
- Infusion

Intention

Perhaps one of the most important steps in blending your herbal remedy is your state of mind. If you are upset with someone or someone has wronged you in some way and you can't stop thinking about it, this is not the time to formulate medicine.

When you are creating your herbal formulas, it is imperative that you are thinking healing thoughts, in a happy frame of mind, without the interference of a TV playing some drama or crime show, hateful music, violent video games, toxic people, hateful people, etc.

A somewhat healing environment needs to be created and that's not to say that if you have children, they shouldn't be around or ANYTHING like that. Children have a high vibration.

What I'm saying is when you are gathering and creating your formulations, you want to have your intention set on healing, imagining the outcome you are striving for, extreme health.

If it's for someone specific, imagine them whole, happy and healthy the whole time while you are preparing it, you can even repeat that while you are formulating it as well as healing thoughts such as; 'I feel better,' 'I grow stronger every day,' 'I enjoy vital health,' and any others that you might think of.

Imagining white light pouring into your formulations from above and filling them with Universal Healing Energy will also potentialize your remedy.

What you wouldn't want to do is think my pain is going away, my pain is gone, my pain has subsided. Every word has a vibration or frequency associated with it, in accordance with The Law of Attraction, we attract that which we focus on. So, we don't want to keep saying pain, or whatever it is that we don't want over and over, we want to say what we do want over and over.

Imagining the desired outcome will ensure the potency of your medicine.

Structured Water

Studies have shown that red blood cells examined under a microscope, indicating that they've lost their electrical charge and are clumped together indicating the possibility of future heart disease, can actually be reversed with a glass of structured water and observed under a microscope. After 12 minutes, the cells become buoyant, slippery, repelling each other and have their electrical charge back.

The best part of this is that you can make structured water by writing the words 'Thank you,' 'Gratitude,' and 'Love' on your glass or water vessel. (Hopefully, you don't drink out of plastic water bottles containing BPA.) In this research, the words that had the most beneficial impact on the water were 'Love' and 'Gratitude.'

Since our bodies are 75% water, it only makes sense to assume that our thoughts can change the cells within our bodies. And our projection can literally change the world around us, so let's set our intention to healing!

The Simpler's Method of Measurements

While there are some folks who are very specific and meticulous in measuring their formulations, there are others who aren't, using a little bit of this and a pinch of that. Whichever way resonates with you is the way to go.

The Simpler's Method breaks recipes into parts instead of cups or ounces or grams. In this way, any herbal recipe can be enjoyed in a cup or on a larger scale. Instead of using cups or ounces, measurements are converted into parts:

- two parts Hibiscus

- one part Dandelion

- three parts Parsley

The Simpler's Method suggests using large quantities of local, mild herbs continuously over a period of time.

Extraction Methods and Dosages:

With room left for Record Keeping- the following lists the procedure for Tinctures, Teas, Decoctions and Infusions:

Extraction	Method + Dosage
Tincture	A tincture is an herbal extraction of alcohol mostly, but glycerin can also be used for children or adults who are sensitive to alcohol. This is usually more potent and powerful than tea because of its concentration. If frequent doses need to be given for treatment when out and about, a tincture is a convenient choice.

Preparation:
Place herbs in a jar
Cover with organic grain alcohol,
(80 - 100% rum, brandy, vodka) can also be used.
Place in a sunny spot allowing the Sun's rays to extract the beneficial compounds into the alcohol. Shake every day for 2-6 weeks, dispersing the molecules into the alcohol while directing your intention towards healing.
Strain
Pour into sterilized dark colored bottles, label.

Dose:
In most cases
1 or 2 dropperful
1 glass of water
Can be taken straight out of the bottle but sometimes they can be strong.
If the symptoms are severe this can be administered up to three times a day.

Extraction	Method + Dosage

For children:
1 dropperful, toddlers ½ of that would suffice.
If the taste is extremely strong, it can be added to juice.

If you're wondering about the alcohol consumption of a child taking the tincture, the amount of alcohol that is actually left is very minute and does not have any effect on the child.

If it still feels uncomfortable, squirt the dropperful into a glass of water and then let sit for 10-20 min. and the alcohol will evaporate.

Tea

Preparation:
Beverage:
1 tsp. herbs
1 cup of water
depending on the plant -
might be necessary to cover during the steeping process to ensure no loss of volatile oils.

But if we are using tea as medicine, larger quantities of herbs would be added.

Making these blends in quart jars and having them on hand is easier than having to make a fresh cup every time for treatments where herbs are being administered throughout the day.

Medicinal:
1 tbs. herbs
1 cup water
Steep for hours or overnight for a stronger remedy
Strain, pour into a sterilized jar, label.

Extraction	Method + Dosage

Decoction

Gently simmering herbs produces a stronger more concentrated infusion. Specific for extracting medicinal compounds found in roots, bark, dried berries, seeds.

Preparation:
Place 4-6 tbs herbs in pot (6-8 if herbs are fresh)
Cover with 1 qt. cold water
Slowly bring to a boil, cover and then simmer gently for about 20-45 minutes
Strain, leave herbs in pot
Pour decoction in quart jar
Pour more hot water onto decocted herbs in pot until there's enough liquid to fill your jar, cap, label.

Infusions

Flowers, leaves and more delicate parts of the plants are usually infused instead of decocted:

Solar Water Infusion

Same directions as for Solar Oil,
But replace with oil with cold water
Place in direct sunlight for several hours

Preparation:
4-6 tbs. herbs
6-8 if herbs are fresh
1 quart almost boiling water
Fill a mason jar with herbs
Pour water or oil over the top of the herbs
Let steep
Cover depending on volatile oil content of plant
Strain, label
Keep in a cool, dark place.
Some highly aromatic roots such as Goldenseal, Ginger and Valerian are often infused instead of decocted.

Extraction   Method + Dosage

Solar Oil Infusion

Preparation:
Fill jar with herbs
Cover with oil of choice
Place in a sunny window
Shake every day infusing with healing intention
Let sit for 2 weeks
Strain
Bottle into sterilized dark colored bottle
Cap with tight fitting lid and label

**Lunar Water
Infusion**

Preparation:
Same directions as for Solar Water,
But place in direct Moonlight for several
hours. Infusion can be left uncovered if
there are not a lot of insects about.

The subtle energies of the Moon casting
Moonbeams and magic upon your herbal formulation brings a spirit of lore and legend.

To boost its magical influence a little
more, infusing under specific moon
phases such as **waxing Moon (grow
ing)** or **waning Moon (decreasing)**
can make a difference.

If you were trying to attract abundance, then
infusion during the waxing Moon would be
optimum, if a decrease in energies such as l
letting go of something, might be better dur
ing the waning Moon.

**Lunar Oil
Infusion**

Same as the Lunar Water, but replace with oil.

Best Oils for Infusion

I love Extra Virgin Olive Oil and Safflower. If you are going to use the oil on your face, care needs to be taken to ensure the oils used are non-comedogenic or that they don't clog pores easily.

Noncomedogenic oils include:
- **Argan**
- **Castor**
- **Evening Primrose**
- **Extra Virgin Olive**
- **Hempseed**
- **Safflower**
- **Shea Butter**

Once the beneficial properties are infused into the oil, it can be used by itself as a moisturizer or added with other oils for an herbal blend or incorporated into a topical product, such as a creme, ointment, salve, etc.

*(Many products contain Grapeseed oil because it is an inexpensive oil, but unless it's organic, I definitely wouldn't use it as grapes are heavily sprayed with pesticides.)

Purity

When heating oils for topical products, never use aluminum pots as they can leach into your medicine, never boil ingredients, never use a microwave or pour hot liquids into plastic. Never use scratched Teflon for heating herbal concoctions (or any other time!)

Glass measuring cups and pots are always the first choice when preparing your formulations, as well as metal measuring spoons, instead of plastic. Plastic really has no place in an Apothecary.

Topicals

The possibilities are endless, there are so many beneficial oils for the skin or that have analgesic, pain relieving properties.

What is the salve for?

- **Skin condition?**
- **Pain?**

Top choices for any kind of skin issues are going to be plant oils high in essential fatty acids, omega-3s, gamma-linolenic acid, antioxidants, etc.

Oils such as:

- **Borage**
- **Evening Primrose**
- **Flaxseed**
- **Hempseed**
- **Rosehip Seed**

are high in essential fatty acids that are crucial for fighting free radicals which can contribute to premature aging, age spots, wrinkles, etc.

Salves

Transforming your herbal oil into a medicinal salve is both easy and fun, taking a very short time.

Salve Preparation

What you'll need:

Herbal oil or combination of oils

Beeswax (if you get beeswax pastilles, it is SO much easier than trying to cut huge blocks)

Vitamin E

Essential oils (only if you want to)

Cutting board (if you don't have pastilles)

Big knife

Glass pot

Rubber spatula

Glass jars or metal tins to pour salve into

Preparation:

1 cup herbal oil

¼ cup beeswax

5 drops of vitamin E oil

Essential oils (optional)

Directions:

On very low heat, melt your beeswax with your herbal oil very slowly, so as to not kill any of the beneficial compounds in the oil.
When melted, take a spoon and stir all the way down to the bottom.
Take the spoon out letting the oil drop off.
Let a few of those droplets fall on a flat surface
Wait for about 5 minutes for them to cool.

Consistency Test:

Check consistency:

- If firm to the touch, but you can still get some oil, that's perfect!

- If it feels hard, like you have to really indent it to get some, then there is too much beeswax. Add a little more oil and test again until desired consistency is reached.

- If it feels completely soft and squishes, then you need to add some more beeswax and test again.

This step is vital to saving you a lot of time and energy. I have not done this in the past and made a huge batch and had to scrape them all out and reheat with more beeswax because they were literally so runny. So, DON'T SKIP THIS STEP!

Add a few drops of vitamin E

Swish around the liquid to distribute the vitamin E

Add essential oils (optional)

|Pour into containers

Put lids over the tops lightly so nothing can fall in but so that the salves can breathe as they set.

Setting Process:

Depending on the size of your container, waiting about an hour should suffice.

Do a test by picking up the container and tilting it to make sure it is solid.

Cap, label.

Muscle Relaxing Salve Preparation:

50-200mg CBD Oil

2 parts Calendula oil

4 parts Arnica oil

6 parts Extra Virgin Coconut oil

2 parts St. John's wort oil

Beeswax

Vitamin E

Equal parts of essential oils:

Lavender

Cedarwood

Sprays

Hydrosols (floral waters) or Herbal Oils:

Two different kinds of topical sprays can be formulated depending on what you are trying to target:

- **Skin issues**

- **Pain relief**

CBD's can restore a healthful glow, regulate sebum production in the skin to prevent dry, flaky skin or oily skin. Full of antioxidants to help our bodies repair the damage from harmful free radicals in our environment. Restore skin cells, rejuvenates your skin, the list goes on, who doesn't need all that?

Pain Relief

Pain relief needs to be addressed by considering plants holding anti-inflammatory properties as well as calming, hormone balancing, antispasmodic, etc. Once you've collected your chosen ingredients blend them well, shake and apply directly onto the affected area.

Because of the way that CBD oil works in the body- reducing cortisol levels, down regulating inflammation, it will be the first choice when trying to treat conditions involving pain. When the body experiences an injury, your brain sends out neurotransmitters to that area with sensitizers, activating your CBD receptors blocks your brain from sending out those neurotransmitters, lessening your perception of the pain while it goes to work repairing any kind of nerve damage or tendon repairs, etc.

Cannabinoids are what our bodies use for pain relief. Our bodies produce cannabinoids but we use them up because of stress in our environment, among other factors. So if you are going through an extremely stressful time, you might need more CBD oil than other days.

Being completely safe, you can adjust your dose by adding a few more drops until the desired results are achieved and then back off when life calms back down a bit. It is nontoxic, non-addictive and has no adverse side effects, unlike any other pain relief script your conventional medical doctor will give you.

If it's dull and achy, you can probably get away with a lower strength, if it gets intense at times then you'd probably want to go with a mid-strength and if it gets extreme, then you will give it all you got!

CBD Dose~

Some folks think dosage has to do with body weight or size but what it really has to do with is the level of Endocannabinoid Deficiency and the severity of the pain or whatever it is you are trying to treat.

We recommend the same dose for a small cat as we would for a 400 lb. man. That being micro-dosing with 2 drops in the morning, under your tongue and 2 drops in the evening, doesn't matter what strength, just go slow, start low.

If you end up needing more, that's fine, but at least you know. Some companies tell you to start with a dropperful or two in the morning and at night and when I say drops instead of dropper, they feel confused. But I always tell folks, if you end up needing that much, that's fine.

But at least you know it instead of starting with so many milligrams. Many of our patients do great with the 4 drops a day, others take 5 drops 3x a day, some take 10 drops in the morning and 10 drops at night. I could tell you to take 1-2 dropperfuls a day, too, there would be a lot of job security in that for me, but if you can get to the same place with a couple drops a day and save your money to go on vacation, wouldn't that be better?

It's very individual, the beauty of it is the ability to play with it with no risk of overdosing. And knowing that stress decreases our cannabinoids, if you are going through an extremely stressful time, you might need to add a few more drops in the morning and or evening, vice versa.

Pain Relief Spray:

CBD Oil~ anywhere from 100mg~up to 500mg depending on the severity of the pain. My products only go up to 200mg for my strongest pain relief product and we've had amazing results, but you can always make them as strong as needed.

CBD oil

4 parts Arnica oil

2 parts St. John's wort oil

6 parts Extra Virgin Olive oil

4 parts Safflower oil

7 drops Cedarwood essential oil

10 drops Rosemary essential oil

5 drops Mint essential oil

3 drops vitamin E oil

Mists

There are many different floral waters available, some of my favorites are Cucumber, Green Tea, Lavender, Rose, Neroli, Rosemary to name a few. These floral waters possess the same properties as the essential oils but on a much gentler, lighter level.

For Aromatherapy purposes, they are perfect carriers for light scents with complementary characteristics to essential oils working synergistically together to balance on either a physical or emotional level. Wonderful for beautifying or shifting the mood.

Generally, not used as medicine for serious conditions as an isolated treatment because of their gentle nature.

To formulate your own, figure out what you are trying to target and find plants with those properties.

General Blending Guidelines:

10 drops Essential Oil

15 ml Hydrosol

Blend hydrosol with your essential oils

I usually use less than this and folks always tell me my formulations are not too strong.

For children:

½ of this amount

Facial Mist Recipe:

1 oz. Lavender hydrosol

10 drops Orange essential oil

Blend together in a sterilized dark colored glass bottle

Cap, label

Labeling

The value that labeling holds is priceless. You might think that there is no way that you could possibly forget what's in that jar, but over time, especially if you are an avid Herbalist with lots of concoctions... just save yourself the time and mental anguish of desperately trying to remember which jar was which.

Not that this has EVER happened to me before, I can just imagine the dilemma before you. 'Ha ha – way too many times!' You would think you'd learn after 30 years, but some habits die hard. Just label it and save yourself the guesswork. Use your brainpower for creating new formulations not trying to remember what the old ones are.

Why Not Mineral Oil?

Mineral oil is pure petroleum. Pure petroleum not only is not recommended for external or internal use, but it also puts a shield on the skin preventing it from breathing. I had a patient with terrible eczema, when I asked her what she was using, she said, Vaseline! That's pure petroleum, no wonder she had eczema!

Considering our skin absorbs 60% of whatever we put on it, if you can't eat it or it's not from a plant or some other ingredient found in the plant kingdom, then you probably should refrain from applying it to your skin.

The number of synthetic ingredients found in personal care products that contain compounds derived from petrochemicals is too long to list here, however, I have included information that I compiled 16 years ago, detailing the toxins in skincare products, what part of your body they affect and the derivative (see Annex B). In this way, you can compare ingredients in the booklet to what is in your medicine chest and if you choose to give yourself cancer then at least you've made an educated decision.

We cannot trust our health in anyone else's hands in these days of Big Pharma and the corruption of cheap fillers. We must educate ourselves about ingredients used in the products we frequently rub into our skin and pick and choose the ones that are best for our health.

Most natural/health food stores, food co-ops, etc. will undoubtedly have these ingredients on their shelves. Products that say, 'organic' even, can have these toxins lurking in their long list of ingredients, you cannot trust that just because it is in a health food store or natural food co-op or says 'organic' that this implies that those ingredients are absent.

Summary ~

In this chapter, we learned the different techniques of extraction that have been used for longer than we can actually perceive. We're beginning to grasp the connectedness of creation.

By now, we understand the concept that what we think actually affects the world around us; and how imperative it is that we direct our intention towards thoughts that are going to benefit us all. Not to get stuck in negative thought patterns reminiscing times we were wronged.

We also understand the importance of directing our attention instead of letting our attention direct us. How we are the masters of our emotions, not that the environment masters our emotions. We learned how easy it could be to affect our health in a positive way by infusing our water with loving intention 'structurizing' it.

We can now utilize an ancient technique when measuring our herbal formulations. We have a clear picture of the differences between the various extraction methods and understand the reasoning behind them. We know how to blend our own preparations and have the key to finding the best plant for our remedy.

Now that we know the effects of microwave radiation on our bodies, we know how vitally important it is to keep it and cell phones as far away from our herbal apothecary and the remedies contained within as possible.

We understand what a waste of our time it would be to not just label it after we make it (learning from my mistakes).

And we are aware of the toxic properties of petrochemicals and how we want to keep them as far away from us and our homes as possible.

Let's just say, 'No' to petrochemicals! Please see Annex for more information about Toxins.

Chapter 5 ~ Targeting Symptoms

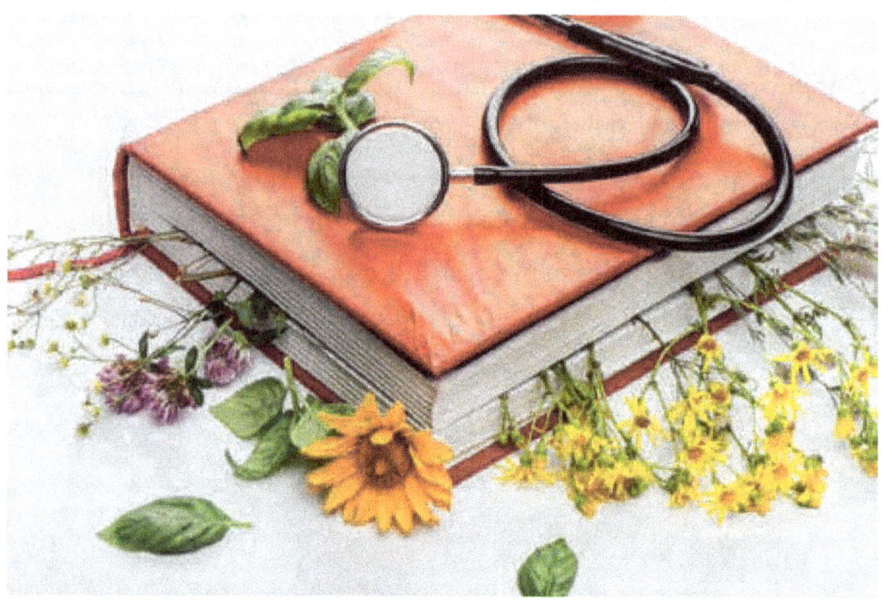

"It is far more important to know what person the disease has than what disease the person has."

— *Hippocrates*

In this chapter, a basic understanding of the importance of stabilization, detoxification and rebuilding and how these methods apply in all situations and are a foundational basis to start your treatment will be given.

The Herxheimer Effect will be identified. The Law of Opposites will be explored as well as an emphasis on research and safety when working with our plant allies. Grasping the toxicity of the diagnostic tests offered is imperative in navigating our decisions guiding us to the safest choices for testing.

A foundation will be laid as to the beauty of Herbal Medicine and the dangers of Black Box Warnings and we'll find out what the leading cause of death in the US is. The dangers of NSAIDs will be investigated as well as the benefits of Energy Medicine and how your thoughts play into not only your personality, your everyday life, but your future as well. We will learn some of the underlying causes of disease that might not be apparent and remedies to rectify those imbalances.

Has your child been diagnosed with a condition or disease? In the end, all diagnoses are just 'terms' that have been used to describe a variety of symptoms, with the exception of cancer. Ultimately, each disease just boils down to 'dis-ease' in the body, including cancer.

We are trying to target specific symptoms and imbalances within the body and restore harmony within the system by moving energy, removing stagnation, nourishing the organs, stimulating circulation, flushing the lymph system, etc.

While some are writing prescriptions containing foreign molecules, we turn not to synthetic molecules but to molecules that the body knows how to synthesize. 'Synthesis over synthetic.'

No Isolated Symptoms

There is never an isolated symptom unless it is the very beginning of disease. The majority of the time, there was something leading up to the illness. If it's an acute (short-term) condition such as a cold or congestion, then not much background is necessary; but for chronic ailments (cancer, emphysema) the root of the cause of dysfunction needs to be located so that it can be removed and then corrected.

Stabilize, Detoxify, Rebuild

Stabilization

With just about any issue the body is experiencing, we need to stabilize its condition, so the body is in a state of homeostasis in which the systems are maintaining stability and functioning properly. We must decrease symptoms enough to manage diet upkeep, begin medicinal tea administration and any compresses or poultices that are needed. Often illness and disease can be a result of an accumulation of toxins in the system, which require elimination.

If the child is too weak or not strong enough to remove them on their own, then the body needs assistance detoxifying. In this case, the first job is to stabilize the condition so that treatment can begin and have efficient absorption. Homeopathic remedies can be administered every 15 minutes during acute situations.

Once the body is stable enough to keep liquids down, nourishing teas can start being administered to build strength. In this state, the patient can relax, eat and conduct themselves without displaying too many symptoms or enduring extreme weakness.

Detoxify

The next objective is detoxification. The body can only withstand so much before it starts experiencing difficulties in managing its normal daily functions. Limit exposure. With too many toxins being introduced, the body becomes stressed and pressured, once you can stabilize it, with the proper nutrients and support needed, it is time to start slowly detoxifying to remove as many of those toxic components as possible.

Herxheimer Effect or the Healing Crisis

Start detox with detoxifying tea blends with any one of these or a combination of Dandelion, Mint, Ginger, Rosemary, Burdock, Astragalus, Echinacea, Green Tea. Administer according to the specific properties in each plant. As the toxins are eliminated, the person could feel worse before better, the importance of detoxifying slowly cannot be stressed enough.

This is called Herxheimer Effect or the Healing Crisis.

- If cancer is the condition being treated, as cancer cells die they accumulate in the blood which can cause an ill feeling.

- If not cancer, the toxins recirculating in the blood as they are removed before they are fully processed by the liver can induce an unpleasant sensation.

During this time the body is detoxing, during this detox, the blood has many toxins running through it causing a variety of symptoms until those compounds are absorbed and processed by the liver. During this detoxing healing process, it is normal for the child to not feel good and sometimes perhaps even feel worse before they feel better. If this is the case then slow down the detox.

While it is a reality, it is not necessary. If the child does not feel good, decrease the quantity or frequency of intervals of administration to slow down the detox and give the body time to process the toxins. Some people say it's necessary, but I don't believe in making children feel worse than they already do even though it's for a good cause. Slowing down the detox process is sometimes more necessary in my opinion than the patient enduring the Healing Crisis.

Distilled Water

Drinking lots of distilled water with a pinch of sea salt attracts impurities from within the body like a magnet and has cleansing properties as well. Oftentimes, detoxification and removing as many toxins as possible in the immediate environment can alleviate many symptoms. After the detox protocol is completed, then beginning to strengthen the body with nervine herbs that build the internal organs can begin.

Rebuilding

This is a vital component in restoring energy and in supporting the growth of new cells. Getting enough rest, in the dark, connecting with our Higher Power, God, Goddess, etc. once a day and filling our bodies full of healing love and energy, plenty of exercise, taking vitamins, enzymes, mushrooms, juicing fresh organic veggies, drinking fresh organic smoothies and toning teas, restoring healthy flora in the gut, maintaining a healing atmosphere, are all THINGS that we can do to increase their quality of longevity.

Treatment

How to treat an individual: Let's say your child has an upset stomach and fever. A tea could be steeped with some Anise to lower the fever and some Mint for the upset stomach. Plants work synergistically together and can be combined in most formulations. Finding the perfect balance of ingredients can sometimes be the tricky part but this is where trial and error comes in.

Other herbs can be added or the amount of herbs can be increased or the frequency of administration can be increased. Think of the symptoms you are trying to treat.

Which one is the most important, or the worst, or causing the harshest symptoms? I would start there, researching herbs to bring relief, then supplement with other herbs that can address symptom management.

One method of practice is to target symptoms or a condition and utilize as many of those plants listed for treating those symptoms in your formulations as possible.

The Law of Opposites

This law teaches us to find plants that produce a similar effect as the one being experienced. Whatever plant would produce those symptoms in a healthy individual when given to a patient experiencing those symptoms results in an absence of those symptoms being presented.

Safety

There are a lot of people giving advice out there. Some is factual, based on research. Other information can be based on beliefs, opinions, or false statements made by misinformed folks. Some information that has been passed down is just directions that were given to children by adults that didn't know better.

Throughout my daughters' childhood, they loved eating chokecherries and green apples (little foragers at heart). Depending on the company we were keeping, they would be told either that chokecherries are poisonous or that eating green apples before they're ripe can make you sick.

And maybe for some, this is true. But when in the company of a local, they'd say, "Those aren't poisonous, we ate those or my grandma made jam out of them!"

Research, Research, Research

So, researching any plant from more than one source can be vital to not only the method of application used for each but which ailments it is best suited or chosen for. There are many plants that can be used for specific ailments but there are specific plants that work better for certain symptoms to maintain the best symptom management.

As an example, if you are suffering from 'congestion' let's say, depending on the symptoms presenting determines how you choose your herbs. Not by disease, what if there was a missed diagnosis? What if it started out as one thing and has progressed into another?

Like from a cold to bronchitis? Are chills present? A fever? For a cough you might choose Elderberry or Wild Cherry Bark, Licorice Root, etc., but if a sore throat was presenting as well then you would add some Slippery Elm for its mucilaginous qualities to soothe and coat the throat.

The beauty of herbal preparations is the ability to utilize many plant compounds in the formulation. What are you trying to target? What symptoms are you trying to treat? What specifically are you trying to do? Having these answers will guide you as to the best choices for your herbal preparations.

The Beauty of Herbal Plant Medicine

The beauty of herbs is the ability to practice trial and error and not jeopardize one's life. In low doses, herbs are safe and can be slightly increased if the desired effect is not achieved. Immediate results should not be expected though. If there's no sign of improvement after 3 days, reevaluate treatment.

Oftentimes, relief can be achieved with mild herbs in large doses with herbal teas for acute conditions but for chronic conditions, sometimes long-term treatment is necessary with stronger herbs.

Sometimes a break in between doses is necessary to let the body function on its own for a week or two and then continue treatment due to the cumulative effects of the herbs on the system, over time.

Take a Break

Herbs producing cumulative effects over time indicating a necessity for a break from treatment for a specific duration required include:

- Goldenseal can affect blood pressure and digestion if taken over extended periods of time.

- Horsetail taken without a break may irritate the kidneys and cause some toxic reactions.

- Kava Kava containing a substance which is stored in the liver and when taken in regular large doses can potentially cause skin eruptions.

If these herbs are being used in treatment, there should be adequate resting periods after any treatment lasting more than six days and when used as directed, they are completely safe.

Intuition

The role that intuition plays in herbal plant medicine is the vital link that was lost. The knowledge that wasn't passed down. The inclination that only our gut can give us. That ancient part of us, the instinctual connection we have to Spirit or Mother Earth that whispers in our ear in a tiny, little plant voice, pick me! It's me, I am the chosen one. I can help restore health and vitality.

As I said, I cannot stress enough the importance of effective research. Always listen to yourself, if you feel the information you are receiving is not accurate, research it instead of believing everything that you hear or read.

Sometimes there are other factors to consider in making and preparing medicinal herbal preparations, such as size, weight, medical issues, contraindications or reactions with other medications, mental state, physical stability, etc.

When my husband was about to start his first five day long chemo treatments that he was scheduled to have every three weeks for three months,

I asked the team of Oncologists at Dartmouth if there was anything that they could suggest to make the impact of the chemo easier on his system when they informed us of all of the side effects: nausea, vomiting, headaches, bone pain, joint pain, neuropathy, mouth sores, ulcers, etc.

Their reply was that it's all how you go into it. If you think, *this is going to be the end of me* it will be. For patients who think, *I'm going to beat this and not let it take me down*, they will have fewer side effects.

This was great information coming from a doctor, that your thoughts play a crucial role in your recovery, which was great for my husband to hear this from someone other than myself.

But at the same time, I knew there had to be some plants that we could incorporate to relieve some of the side effects on a physical level too. I wasn't really sure which ones exactly, but I knew enough to know that Echinacea would probably be one to boost his immune system.

And I could think of others for nausea but I didn't really have any first-hand experience with chemo or cancer. I said to my husband, "I just need to research it and see if there's some herb like Astragalus (of which I had never worked with before) that would help increase your white blood cells and ease the side effects."

Like I said Astragalus was not an herb that I had any experience with and I don't even know why I said it. But in my research, it turned out that it was a powerful ally to have on our side. I learned that it is used in Asia, given to patients who are undergoing chemo treatments.

Why did it pop into my head? That, I can't explain, but it was one of the best herbs for the remedy we were seeking at the time. So, sometimes intuition plays a vital role in the best herbal allies chosen for a particular treatment.

Remember to listen to yourself! If a plant pops into your mind when you think of a specific ailment, symptom or person, that is unfamiliar to you, research its properties. It may turn out to be your wisest choice for a specific ailment or a welcome addition to your preparation.

Diagnostic Tests

Sometimes tests are helpful. Unfortunately, many of the tests in Orthodox Medicine either leave toxic residues or even worse. There's a chance you might not live through it. Why do you think they ask you to sign a release saying you know it could cause a stroke, heart attack or even death? But if the effects of the tests are so toxic that they are comparable to the disease or even worse, then are they really beneficial?

In other words, if injecting radioactive dye that will never leave your system and is carcinogenic (toxic, cancer-causing) is an option, then maybe a wiser choice might be to identify symptoms and find herbs that either diminish the effects or that strengthen the system.

Often these tests are called 'Routine Procedures' implying that there is no danger, but when you look at the statistics, they are not that high in your favor.

Non-Invasive Tests

If there is a non-invasive test that you can have, then, sure, why not? Such as a blood test to see if there's any sign of an infection, or a vitamin test to check your B12 levels or Vitamin D. But what if you didn't have anything that bad wrong with you and you ended up with a stroke, perforated bowel, heart attack or dying?

The treatment should not exceed the disease! I'm not sure in what book it says that's ok. Below are links to another test that they have come up with that has 92% accuracy and it's a stool sample. Why risk death if you're trying to avoid it?

Sometimes a test can be helpful in knowing the direction of your herbal treatment or to know if it's working, such as a blood test for platelet count, white blood cell production, infections, etc. But only if it's not risking the end of your life.

Nothing could be as bad or as uncomfortable as that. Pharmaceutical companies and doctors love to say that the risks of the disease outweigh the side effects of the medication and procedures, but is that really the case when death or stroke is a side effect? What could be worse than that? Doctors take a Hippocratic Oath to do no harm, don't they?

Some helpful links:

- http://m.startribune.com/mayo-offers-alternative-to-colonoscopy-thoughit-has-its-own-ick-factor/250982021/
- https://www.cologuardtest.com/landing?gclid=EAIaI-QobCh
MI0oy0-
oa2wIVFiWBCh3tAAW7EAAYASAAEgJo0_D_BwE

Pharmaceutical Medications

What is wrong with your medication? Over 125,000 Americans die each year from properly prescribed medications. In the US, we are kind of on our own. We don't really have an organized regulatory body ensuring quality on products being offered for personal care or pharmaceuticals.

With hundreds of thousands of people dying every year from properly prescribed medications, meaning they took it as prescribed and died. Not to mention, the billions of dollars that was given out to vaccine injured families, it is clear that no one has your family's back or their interests in mind. It is what's in the stakeholders' pockets that's being prioritized.

That's why if someone tries to prescribe something for you or your child in a white coat, remember they are just 'practicing medicine.' What was OK for one might not be for you or your family with so many different variables to take into account. No one knows what's best for your family other than you.

Always read pharmaceutical information thoroughly so you know what to be aware of and what to avoid. This is where the beauty in herbal medicine lies. While of course there are toxic plants, most herbs trigger healing even in minute quantities but do not cause harm until unlikely levels for use are reached.

Properly Prescribed

"About 2,460 people per week are estimated to die from drugs that were properly prescribed and that's based on detailed chart reviews of hospitalized patients," says Light, who is a professor of comparative health policy at Rowan University School of Osteopathic Medicine in Stafford, New Jersey.

That does not include overdoses or using prescribed drugs unintended, that is PROPERLY PRESCRIBED, meaning you used it as instructed following your doctor's directions.

Bring In Backup

If we've tried every plant we can and for some reason we are just not seeing any improvement than it might be time to bring in back up, but it's what kind of backup you call in that can be the difference between life and death.

Alternative Practitioners

Seek out a Naturopathic Doctor in your area or a Holistic Health Care Practitioner, Homeopath, Functional Medicine Doctor, Clinical Cannabiniod Clinician, Chiropractor, Acupuncturist, etc. Acupuncture is another healing modality that many have never tried.

If you are experiencing discomfort and 'nothing' seems to be helping, this could be due to energetic blockages along your Meridians or Energy Pathways that run through the body. The gentle yet effective pressure from Acupuncture needles can be just the remedy when all else fails. Acupressure is similar, not involving the use of needles.

Kinesiology

Personally, I go see my Kinesiologist, her name is Dr. Francine and she is amazing! Kinesiologists understand the silent art of reading your bodies subtle impulses indicating what it prefers. It's a way of reading the bodies language. I always go see her if I ever feel like I have any health issues and direct my daughters to do the same. Oftentimes, they can pick up imbalances within your system that Orthodox Medicine's tests cannot because the imbalance has not progressed to that level of disease, yet.

When my husband was undergoing treatment, we went to her and she advised how many capsules his body indicated was necessary for each supplement.

This was invaluable because many of them were far off from the recommendation on the bottle, his body required much more. She also had 'standardized supplements' that she prescribed for him.

Why Not Just Use The Plant?

Humans have been referring to plants for assistance with disease within the body for thousands of years, since there were humans and plants. Many medications today are derived from some molecule in the plant kingdom that they tried to duplicate in the lab because they recognize the potential benefits of those plant compounds.

'Why not just use the plant?' you ask. You cannot patent a plant and charge a lot of money for the medicine derived from it because you didn't create the plant. If you can duplicate that molecule in the lab, you can patent it, say it works for such and such diseases and make bank on it from any individual suffering from such and such disease.

Many people say, 'we are living longer today than we ever did and that is thanks to the breakthroughs in modern medicine with all of their procedures and new medications.' Which sounds good unless you do the research and find that most of a medication's side effects can cause so much damage and wreak so much havoc on your body that you can actually die! The FDA does not have your back, so don't think for a second, 'well those drugs are regulated.'

All of their medications have adverse effects on the body by stopping the body's natural reactions to try and restore balance in the system. Many of them cause nausea because your body is trying to rid itself of the toxic substance you just put in it. Many of them block your body from producing melatonin which is necessary for your optimum sleep processes.

Some of them block cholesterol, which is your body's natural anti-inflammatory agent, your body produces it to patch damage in your arteries, if you have too much, curbing your diet is one way to reduce your cholesterol, not by trying to keep it lower with medication and continuing to eat foods that are causing inflammation and damage triggering your cholesterol, fever reducers - your body is doing its job trying to burn out an invader.

After the body breaks a sweat with a fever, that sweat has natural antibacterial, antibiotic properties to it that can kill staph! Let your body do its job.

No Research Showing NyQuil Increasing Recovery Time

When the body produces a fever, it's an effort to kill some kind of pathogen such as bacteria or a virus. If we stop the body from producing these defense mechanisms, we not only are stopping our body from fighting with its natural defenses.

We take Benadryl or Tylenol to lower a fever, which only inhibits the immune system even further with its compounds that the liver has to filter and tries to process on top of fighting an invader or trying to keep them at bay.

Obviously, too high of a fever is very dangerous. But there's lots of research showing that cold medicines do not decrease the length or duration of a cold. There is no research showing that taking NyQuil or any other OTC medications has any effect on increasing the recovery time.

On a molecular level, our bodies can only process that which comes from the natural world. Our bodies were not made to process all of the chemicals, vaccines and medications we inject into it. It has nowhere to go, it sits somewhere, causes inflammation and then disease.

Whatever medication you are on, there is a plant that can do it better! Take back your health, don't just stop taking your prescription by any means, many of them cause more adverse effects if you discontinue use without tapering it off.

If your issue is high blood pressure, there are plants for that, thyroid dysfunction, there are plants for that, cancer, there are plants for that- no matter what kind of disease it is, heart disease, there are plants for that, diabetes, there are plants for that, neurological disorders, there are plants for that, pain, etc.

Black Box Warning

Are you familiar with the Black Box Warning in your pharmaceutical medication box? Most people don't even read it. Antidepressants include them. There are two lists of side effects for medications, the ones that are life-threatening such as stroke, heart attack, kidney failure, liver damage, thyroid dysfunction, hemorrhaging, death and the ones that are not, such as nausea, headache, vomiting, muscle pain, inflammation, shortness of breath, dizziness, etc.

When the list of side effects is larger for the life-threatening side effects than the less serious side effects, it has what's known as a 'Black Box Warning.' How can something even be offered to us that can cause such dysfunction within our bodies? How can we even agree to that?

Unless Assisted Suicide is a law, I don't know how it could even be legal much less ethical to prescribe a drug to someone with such life-threatening dangers. What could be so bad that it would be worth risking any of those severe side effects?

It has become such the norm that people don't even think anything about the side effects, anymore. But they're not even side effects, these are DIRECT effects of the medications, the side effects are any possible BENEFIT you might experience.

Non-Steroidal Anti-Inflammatories (NSAIDS)

As an example, has anyone ever read on a bottle of Tylenol, Ibuprofen, Advil that it could cause a heart attack, stroke, GI bleed? And not after prolonged use, the first time, there's a possibility that this could happen with no warning. GI bleeds happen more often than people think. According to Dr. Sunil Pai, '100,000 people a year go to the hospital from taking NSAIDS, 22,000 people die a year from taking these drugs.

From 1984 to 2009 almost 300,000 people died from taking nonsteroidal anti-inflammatories. That's more people than died in the Revolutionary War, more than the War of 1812, Mexican American War, Spanish American War, World War One, Korean War, Vietnam, Persian Gulf and Iraq and Afghanistan combined.'

Just to give you an idea of how many innocent lives Big Pharma is destroying with their poisons. These are people who just were experiencing pain maybe from a golf injury or twisted the wrong way, picked up their grandchild when they shouldn't have, were shoveling snow, innocent people that trusted that if a product was sold 'over-the-counter' that it meant that it was safe to take.

And there's now proof that NSAIDs deteriorate your joints. After 2 years, you can see visible changes on x-rays demonstrating that it actually makes arthritis worse.

Massage

Gentle massage is always a great way of relaxing a child's body and moving toxins around so they can be processed, increasing circulation, etc.

Note: Not recommended for lymphoma patients, massage can metastasize the cancer. Gentle bouncing on a small trampoline some refer to as a 'rebounder' is a great way to flush the lymphatic system for patients or others suffering from lymphatic system disorders.

With the varying number of massage techniques ranging from Swedish to Thai to Deep Tissue, Shiatsu, Shamanic, etc. all known to increase vitality including gentle breathing techniques to light to moderate stretching techniques such as Feldenkrais, which is not massage, not Yoga, not Tai Chi or Qi Gong, but a specific way of stretching. Tai Chi, Qi Gong and Yoga are all light movement techniques used around the world to stimulate the energy of the body, unblocking Chakras, clearing energy centers and affecting more than just the physical level but the astral body as well.

Chakras

When we experience blockages in our energy centers it can cause energy to stagnate. What do we mean by energy centers? We have seven Chakras that we will speak of now for the purpose of this book. These energy centers are found along our spine and are similar to spinning vortexes of energy. They are each correlated with various organs and systems in our body. When they become blocked, we can see a deterioration of energy in those areas corresponding to these energy centers.

The beauty of herbs is that they not only affect the physical body, but they have an obvious, noticeable, recordable effect on the energetic body as well. Some disease stems from a physical imbalance, but much disease begins on an energetic level before it reaches the physical body.

This confirms the importance of stress relieving and Mindfulness Techniques to clear away negative energies or blockages imperative to optimum health. We cannot only address the physical body and expect to affect the whole by ignoring the energetic body.

The body translates emotions into physical chemicals and hormones in the body that are either causing stress sending the body into 'Fight or Flight' or that are reducing cortisol and other stress hormones such as adrenaline.

These hormones can be helpful when needed for short-term stressful situations but when the body lives in this constant state, it can interfere with neurotransmission of chemicals needed for vital health.

Neurotransmitters

These are sent from the brain to the internal organs with messages for the body to signal secretion and suppression of specific hormones. It is a lock and key system. If the brain cannot produce the correctly sized and shaped neurotransmitter, it will not fit into the receptor. So then the messages that the brain is trying to send will not make it through.

Then the hormones or chemicals that should have been suppressed or produced weren't and these neurotransmitters just keep circulating because they don't fit anywhere. When these messages do not make it to where they were intended, it creates imbalances in the body.

These imbalances in turn create emotions and feelings that could be avoided if Mindfulness Techniques such as Yoga, meditation, Qi Gong, Tai Chi, etc. were employed by allowing our bodies to resist the urge to always be active and engaged in our environment which can cause stress and ill health.

Emotions: Are They the Root Cause of Your Disease?

They say no one really knows the role our emotions play in disease, but we can see how important they are in healing as well as the possible root cause when we realize what kind of chemical reactions our emotions can cause within our bodies. Our thoughts literally change the physiology within our bodies. This isn't belief, this isn't opinion, it is science.

Chinese Medicine Wheel

We now understand the ancient wisdom that Asia has bestowed upon us correlating specific emotions to certain organs:

- **Fear - Kidney/Adrenal/Sex Organs**

- **Worry - Stomach/Spleen/Pancreas**

- **Anger - Liver/Gallbladder**

- **Anxiety - Heart/Small Intestine**

Immune Boosting

Some folks enjoy supreme health, almost taking it for granted, but for some, the idea of optimum immune function seems out of reach. However, if we look further into what 'proper immune function' even means, we might be better able to apply these principles into our everyday life so that it isn't some drastic lifestyle change, or huge purge of everything close to us, but rather a consistent stream of constant choices that steadily lead us on the path to a healthier more resilient immune system.

First of all, where is your immune system, even? Do you know? I bet one guess might be your white blood cells, which is a good one, but there's so much more to it. Your tonsils are part of your immune system sitting as tiny reservoirs of white blood cells attacking any invaders that enter through the mouth before they can reach the internal organs.

That's why when doctors recommend removing them, it's not always necessarily the wisest option and other possibilities or underlying factors should be investigated before the removal. In the 1960s when it became popular to remove children's tonsils, those children had more cavities than the children who still had their tonsils, not having that protection.

Briefly, our thymus gland, under the breastbone, produces T-cells, which are the most active and most daring lymphocytes or fighter white blood cells, there are several types of white blood cells. Helper T-cells identify invaders and stimulate the production of other immune cells located in the spleen and lymph nodes.

Other important areas of lymph tissue throughout the body include the appendix and throughout the intestinal tract. 80% of our immune system lies in our intestinal tract, which explains why having healthy bacteria (probiotics) in the correct concentrations to ensure health and longevity is vital.

Dangerous viruses such as HIV have some DNA, although not the complete molecule, so they invade a healthy cell, stealing its DNA and use it to propagate and increase in number.

This host cell can be a blood cell or any cell in the body, eventually, this parasitic action results in the cell becoming 'bleached out' by having its nutrients expended causing it to rupture and spew the virus into healthy tissue which it continues to invade. Not only limited to autoimmune diseases or cancer.

Imbalances

Symptoms of poor immune function include:

- **dark circles under the eyes**
- **cravings**
- **sinus problems**
- **joint and muscle dysfunction**
- **headaches**
- **coughing**
- **rashes**
- **emotional behavior problems**
- **mood swings**
- **respiratory problems**
- **food sensitivities**
- **hay fever**

All of the above are signs of an immune system whose function is being diminished by some imbalance that either originates **chemically, physically, or electromagnetically**.

Improving immune function includes many different facets and is not limited to any one choice, action or medication. So many different factors contribute to immune boosting and optimum immune function such as increasing white blood cells, increasing available energy in the body, removing blockages, removing causes contributing to diminished immune function, improving circulation, detoxing the liver, eliminating factors contributing to increased stress levels, lowering stress levels, lowering cortisol and adrenaline levels, improving digestion, absorption and bioavailability of nutrients, purifying the blood, improving mental clarity, practicing Mindfulness Techniques, gratitude, forgiveness, increasing serotonin and oxytocin or love chemical hormones, strengthening your macrophage, balancing your gut biome, etc.

Chemical Imbalance

This could either be food related or literally chemically related such as toxins you are exposing your body to in the form of personal care products, cleaning agents, air fresheners, chemicals you work with such as at a salon or garage, etc. Something as simple as not getting enough vitamins and nutrients can play an integral role in wellness.

Nutritional deficiencies can cause all kinds of biochemical reactions in the body. A good, organic multivitamin, food derived, might be a wise, healthy choice to optimize immune function and what an easy place to start?

So, if for some reason you didn't eat all of your recommended daily allowances of vitamins and minerals for the day, you know that your body is not lacking in the vital compounds required.

Physical Imbalance

Could stem or originate from some trauma, accident, abuse, blockage, etc. and can usually be corrected by some form of Chiropractic care, not always cracking.

Electromagnetic Imbalances

Includes but not limited to cell phones, Wi-Fi, EMF's (electromagnetic fields) such as emanating from appliances, microwaves, electronics, Smart meters, cell towers, 5G, etc.

What are Immune-Compromising Lifestyle Choices?

Well, to name a few:

- **Diet**

- **Microwaves**

- **Technology**

- **Environment**

- **Personal Care Products**

Some we have control over and can change...some...not so much.

Which is all the more reason to make the necessary changes where you can... because there are some choices we make that are unavoidable, like getting in a car every day, not much choice there if you need to work or take your children to school or go buy groceries. But, do you have to choose to drink something that will take the paint off of a car is the question? (Referring to Coke)

If we look at each of those very briefly:

Diet: The SAD (Standard American Diet) is actually disease causing, what with the GMOs that are not even allowed in other countries, high fructose corn syrup, sugar, soda, etc. Follow this link to find out more: Genetic Roulette, by Jeffrey Smith is a shocking eye opening documentary that explains it all.

https://www.youtube.com/watch?v=7sUNxX0OxP8

Microwaves: When food is cooked in a microwave, it actually changes the cells within the food into carcinogens...aka cancer-causing! How can it be called food if it causes cancer? Food is supposed to nourish the body...sustain life. Here is a link to review:

UPDATE: When this book was written the link was up, it has since been taken down as Google is removing whatever they don't agree with it seems.

But I was able to find a snippet of the article on Duck Duck Go another search engine:

https://www.huffpost.com/entry/microwave-　cancer_b_684662?guccounter=1&guce_refer-rer=aHR0cHM6Ly93d3cuZ29vZ2xlLmNvbS8&guce_refer-rer_sig=AQAAAHn7b7dmC022e5U9pApm1u_0zRsRd1WjvdriVfDFQJbl_09zbgJhRm46Y_1lw8HJvqu9nGe3Aw

7ldXi7MaU13wREJbGF8TlBGk6hHmFQgbKkvMM7v24s3DYQetS5
AcSM7UyAvFzTPMi0Mmj4hRtO0ncKR22 UoZljvHq4sWdO-Qs

Here is another helpful article:

https://naturalsociety.com/microwaves/

Technology: The amount of time spent with your device in your hand, on your person or near your head while sleeping is enough to cause cancer. Here is a link to review:

181022_EMF Studies from Powerwatch.pdf

Environment: Depending on where we live, we could be drinking polluted water...chlorinated, fluoridated water, etc. We could be breathing toxic pollution from factories nearby, exhaust, perfumes, bleach, cleaning products, etc. We can be in close proximity to cell phone towers, 5G, power plants, electrical stations, etc.

Skincare Choices: Our skin is our largest organ, absorbing 60% of what we put on it. Most products sold contain toxic, cancer-causing chemicals because there are no regulations on body care products in the US at this time.

Even products labeled organic and natural, sold in health food stores and natural food co-ops, can still contain these chemicals. 'Natural' labeling doesn't really mean anything, anymore. See Annex B for more information about toxins.

We see that many of the choices we make in a day can compromise our immune system. If we are not immune-compromised, we might not even notice. But if we are, these should be avoided at all costs. Our immune system has to be what cures us, not medication.

When my husband was undergoing treatment, we received the little booklet that goes along with chemo about your blood and what symptoms would indicate what feelings, for instance, low red blood count would mean you would feel sluggish and tired. I realized how when we feel certain symptoms it is because our body is lacking in something.

Which usually always goes back to something that Nature can provide. Do you need to boost your white blood cell count? Lower your blood pressure, increase your energy, increase your appetite? Fight infection? Improve circulation? Support a healthy metabolism? Detoxify? Absorb vital nutrients? Whatever it is, Nature can help.

Entertainment

But for your child's entertainment, there is a reason they say 'laughter is the best medicine.' Our bodies secrete certain hormones that stimulate growth and that make us receptive when we are happy, laughing, enjoying life. Sure, we may not be able to change the world around us, bad things might happen, but we can change the world within us, what we bring in, what we listen to, watch, what we focus on.

If what they focus on is drama, death and dying, trauma, constant sadness, living in a state of dread because of what they choose to 'entertain' themselves with, then how can we really expect them to ever feel better when they're not experiencing much joy? If they surround their self with shows full of depression and anxiety and can't figure out why they don't feel good, hopefully reading this will help!

A Little about Ions

Ever wonder why you just seem to feel better in Nature? Let's say near a river, lake, the ocean or a mountain? Well, if we talk a little bit about negative ions and positive ions, we might begin to understand why this is not just a belief, but a fact.

Positive Ions

Every living cell in our bodies has an electrical current in it, as I keep reiterating, we are literally vibrating at a specific frequency individual to each human body. Our magnetic field is made of both positive and negative ions. Positive ions are created by cell phones, TVs, computers, Wi-Fi, etc. and can adversely affect our mood. Overexposure to these ions can create a multitude of physical symptoms such as depression, fatigue, lethargy, etc.

Negative Ions

Abundant negative ions are found in Mother Nature when water is in motion such as after a rain shower or by the beach with the waves crashing or near a rushing river, even fountains. They are generated in large quantities as air molecules break apart from moving water.

This would explain why you feel so good after a shower, because you are creating your own negative ions. Air movement (wind), Sunlight, plants and radioactive decay of noble gases also naturally create them. Negative ions are lighter and smaller and more likely to become airborne, positive ions, being heavier tend to fall to the ground. This would explain why it feels so good to be outside because it is literally GOOD FOR YOU!

Sick Building Syndrome

Ever heard of Sick Building Syndrome? Our homes today are so tight that little or no outside air can get in, our heating and air conditioning systems can produce positive ions. Too much time indoors can literally zap your energy and make you feel ill, between your phone and all the other electronic devices in your home.

Just to give you an idea, the ocean is reported to have tens of thousands of negative ions while the average home, office, building may contain a few hundred to none.

Salt Lamps

These lamps are always a great way to increase the negative ions in your indoor space whether it's an office or home. Not only is the soft, illuminating light emanating from them relaxing and calming, but they are actually air purifiers!

So, open the windows, go outside, get a little or big, even, fountain in your house, we have a cute Buddha one in ours right next to our Salt

Lamp. It's so basic, costs nothing, no prescription needed and you could feel better...it's a no brainer! Open the windows, get outside, put down your phone!

Is Fluoride a Neurotoxin?

... Then why is it in our toothpaste and drinking water?

There are actually dentists who are advocating and trying to bring awareness to this serious issue. Yes, fluoride is absolutely a neurotoxin. What does that mean? A neurotoxin, the definition is a poison that works on the nervous system. It impedes the brain's development, neuro is associated with nerves and toxin generally means poisonous, dangerous, life-threatening. I am attaching many resources for folks to do their own research.

It is hard to believe that we are having our children put something in their mouth and brush their teeth with it that says **if you swallow more than a pea sized amoun**t call poison control...at some point we have to think for ourselves.

Some people say it is a nutrient, first off, let's straighten that out, it is NOT a nutrient.

Neurotoxin

Even more importantly, fluoride has been identified as a developmental neurotoxin that impacts short-term and working memory and contributes to rising rates of attention-deficit hyperactive disorder and lowered IQ in children.

Many of these studies have found harm at levels within the range, or precariously close to, the levels that millions of American children receive regularly. In all, there are more than 300 animal and human studies demonstrating fluoride can cause:

- Brain damage, especially when coupled with iodine deficiency or excessive levels of aluminum

- Reduced IQ

- Impaired ability to learn and remember

- Neurobehavioral deficits such as impaired visual-spatial organization

- Impaired fetal brain development

Impact of Fluoride on Neurological Development in Children

"Fluoride seems to fit in with lead, mercury, and other poisons that cause chemical brain drain," Grandjean says.

In an excerpt from the Harvard University news article which you can find by following this link:

https://www.hsph.harvard.edu/news/features/fluoride-childrens-health-grandjeanchoi/

'The average loss in IQ was reported as a standardized weighted mean difference of 0.45, which would be approximately equivalent to seven IQ points for commonly used IQ scores with a standard deviation of 15. Some studies suggested that even slightly increased fluoride exposure could be toxic to the brain. Thus, children in high fluoride areas had significantly lower IQ scores than those who lived in low fluoride areas. The children studied were up to 14 years of age, but the investigators speculate that any toxic effect on brain development may have happened earlier, and that the brain may not be fully capable of compensating for the toxicity.'

UPDATE: Another link that has gotten removed, last year when this book was originally written, these articles could be found but have since been removed by Google. Refer to this article by Dr. Axe for the same info describing the reality about this situation:

https://draxe.com/health/is-fluoride-bad-for-you/

The American Cancer Society has this information on their website: 'The EPA has also set a secondary standard of no more than 2.0 mg/L to help protect children (under the age of 9) from *dental fluorosis*.' In this condition, fluoride collects in developing teeth, preventing tooth enamel from forming normally. This can cause permanent staining or pitting of teeth.

Some of the controversy about the possible link stems from a study of lab animals reported by the US National Toxicology Program (NTP) in 1990. The researchers found 'equivocal' (uncertain) evidence of cancer-causing potential of fluoridated drinking water in male rats, based on a higher than expected number of cases of osteosarcoma (a type of bone cancer). There was no evidence of cancer-causing potential in female rats or in male or female mice.

Endocrine-Disrupting Chemical

Dr. Mercola reports, 'Scientific investigations have revealed fluoride is an endocrine-disrupting chemical, and have linked it to the rising prevalence of thyroid disease, which in turn can contribute to obesity, heart disease, depression, and other health problems. In fact, in the 1950s and 1960s, fluoride was used as a drug to lower thyroid activity in patients with over-active thyroid.'

Osteosarcoma

'Most of the concern about cancer seems to be around osteosarcoma. One theory on how fluoridation might affect the risk of osteosarcoma is based on the fact that fluoride tends to collect in parts of bones where they are growing. These areas, known as *growth plate*s, are where osteosarcomas typically develop. The theory is that fluoride might somehow cause the cells in the growth plate to grow faster, which might make them more likely to eventually become cancerous.

The US Environmental Protection Agency (EPA) has set a maximum amount of fluoride allowable in drinking water of 4.0 mg/L. Long-term exposure to levels higher than this can cause a condition called skeletal fluorosis, in which fluoride builds up in the bones. This can eventually result in joint stiffness and pain and can also lead to weak bones or fractures in older adults,' according to the American Cancer Society. You can read more about that here:

https://www.cancer.org/cancer/cancer-causes/water-fluoridation-and-cancerrisk.html

UPDATE: This is another article that has been taken down since the original writing of this book. But you can refer to the link below for some of the same info:

https://www.cancer.org/content/dam/CRC/PDF/Public/7030.00.pdf

Another expert who spoke out about the concerns of the safety of fluoride is John Colquhoun, a dentist in New Zealand who was appointed Principal Dental Officer of Auckland, New Zealand's largest city. Dr. Colquhoun, once passionately pro-fluoridation, reexamined the facts and studies available on fluoridation and wrote an explanation of his staunchly anti-fluoridation stance in *Perspectives in Biology and Medicine* in 1997.

Medicating Our Public Water Supply?

We are one of the only countries that adds medication to the public water supply. If it is for tooth decay, then that would be a medicine.

Most countries would consider asking consent before a mass medicating. On the FDA's website, it is classified as medicine, so if that is the case, people should have some say whether they want to be medicated, wouldn't you agree??

For us Vermonters, with so much fresh, clean water, this might not hit home, but for people who are hooked into a municipal water supply, it is serious because your children are not only ingesting fluoride in their toothpaste but also in their water, absorbing large quantities when bathing along with chlorine.

Teenagers are beginning to show signs of over fluoridation in these municipalities that fluoridate. So not only is the fluoride not lowering the rates of tooth decay, but it is actually detrimental to these poor children's teeth.

Poison

Fluoride is actually a poison so how did it end up in our water? Rachel Hall, a dentist from Australia, explains, 'The fluoride in our water started out as an industrial waste byproduct of aluminum production. In the early 1900s, manufacturers dumped fluoride in landfills and rivers until it was discovered to be poisoning nearby crops and making livestock sick.

This was a problem as it meant the aluminum manufacturers who had no means to dump their by-products had to find another way to get rid of this fluoride waste.

In 1931, researchers found a link between fluoride and tooth decay so the aluminum company who set up their own research institute sent a dentist to study remote towns with naturally occurring high concentrations of calcium fluorides in their water wells.

Through the studies the dentist found a link between high fluoride in drinking water and mottled tooth enamel – called dental fluorosis. This mottling is caused by damage to the enamel formation from having too much fluoride.

The aluminum research center called the Mellon Institute, aimed to support industries. They produced research showing asbestos was safe and did not cause cancer, for example. The research was done to help companies find ways to get rid of their toxic waste.

One of their scientists in 1939 contended that rather than removing fluoride from food and water they should allow a level of contaminate of 1 part per million as it would prevent dental decay.

The Mellon Institute went on to produce reports that assured fluoride was non-toxic and would be beneficial to add to the drinking water for healthy teeth. These reports were supported by the American Dental Association.'

Is this not similar to the tobacco and sugar industries sponsoring their own research to show no harm?

Drowsiness, Mental Confusion and Lethargy

In the mid to late 1940s, a group from the US Health Department was set up to look at the effects of fluoride. These studies were classified and not released for a long time after, showed that fluoride was detrimental to living organisms with effects on the central nervous system leading to drowsiness, mental confusion and lethargy.

Violent Poison to all Living Tissue

Fluoride was defined in 1950 as a violent poison to all living tissue. It was also stated that continuous ingestion of non-fatal doses cause permanent inhibition of growth and the use of fluoride containing toothpastes and internal medicaments is not justified. You can read the whole article at:

https://evolvedental.com.au/fluoride-part-1-fluoride-end-drinking-water/

UPDATE: Guess what? This one has been removed also since the original writing of this book, but I found many other ones that you can link to here:

https://www.evolvedental.com.au/blog/category/fluoride/

Either way, the question is and remains, "Why are we putting an industrial waste chemical into our drinking water and in our toothpaste and then telling our children not to swallow it or not even telling them because we assume that the toothpaste we are using isn't poison or they couldn't sell it to us?"

But go and look on your toothpaste tube and you will see it says to call poison control if more than a pea sized amount is swallowed. If you are not supposed to swallow it, then why is it in our drinking water? And why are there such awful cases of tooth decay in underprivileged areas that have been fluoridated since the 1950s?

Those children's teeth should be getting better after 50+ years of fluoridating not so bad that dental health officials are describing decay that is unexplainable. But don't believe me; go do your own research. I've given you lots of resources. Maybe for 2020, our motto can be, 'Keep your waste out of my child's mouth!'

Additional Resources

http://fluoridealert.org/ http://www.nofluoride.com/

UPDATE: Another one taken down since the original writing of this book.

Try this one from that same source:

http://fluoridealert.org/issues/health/
https://iaomt.org/
https://iaomt.org/resources/fluoride-facts/

Essential Oils - Gifts of the Gods

Many people have heard of essential oils, some have seen them, some have tried them; many have used them, but didn't really understand their structure, their complexity, their beauty, their diversity, their efficacy, their similarities, their many applications.

"The enormous vital energy that radiates from pure essential oils and the weakness of synthetic oils can be measured with a divining rod or Geiger counter. The results are similar to those shown in Kirlian photography and other related methods. A synthetic oil is a dead product. In the eyes of holistic practitioners, it should not be used for healing, strengthening, or health promoting purposes."

— Susanne Fischer-Rizzi
(Author of Complete Aromatherapy Handbook)

Used For Over 5000 Years

Sometimes people turn to essential oils for their cleaning needs, sometimes for personal care, but they actually are so much more than that, they are actual plant medicine. They have been used for over 5000 years; they are mentioned in the Bible over 300 times. They are mentioned in other ancient texts all over the world, from Egypt to Greece to China, etc.

They were the medicine that people used and turned to, their extraction process might have differed and they might have been using a slightly different product, but either way, they were using the life essence of the plants, extracted, concentrated and applying it. Hippocrates alone documented over 200+ herbs.

That's not just their past record, there are over 17,000 studies, today, proving their efficacy. More than 1000 physicians use essential oils in their practices today, in France, alone. Their popularity is returning after a kind of a fog has been lifted, prescription medicine users are learning the adverse side effects of their medications and are turning to more natural remedies for alternatives.

Some side effects might be experienced by essential oils, but they are not adverse, is the difference. Like any other substance, essential oil users' bodies differ and what is fine for one might not be for another and if not administered properly, can cause adverse side effects.

But if used properly, such as diluting oils that should not be applied without carrier oils and remembering less is more, performing patch tests, the effects and results are amazing in how they support, strengthen and tone the body with a synergy that cannot be found by conventional, prescribed or OTC over-the-counter drugs.

Blood Brain Barrier

Beginning with your brain is a great place to start. Some essential oils have compounds in them such as sesquiterpenes, tiny molecules that allow them to pass through the blood/brain barrier supporting the brain, which in turn supports the rest of the body, directly, as most signals originate in the brain. Some also have the ability to reduce the perception of pain, they trigger neurotransmitters in your brain to secrete certain hormones specific to the essential oil's properties.

Brain Cancer and Sesquiterpenes

Frankincense, for example, the sesquiterpenes passing through the blood brain barrier cause apoptosis or cellular suicide to cancer cells, which is a welcome alternative to radiation for those suffering from brain cancer.

Chemistry

Each essential oil's chemistry makeup relates with the body in a different way. It is a specific molecule or chain of molecules that create different reactions to support harmony in the body. Some essential oils have smaller molecules allowing them to absorb quickly into the bloodstream.

Transdermal Application

Applying essential oils on thin skin ensures a speedy absorption rate. Some can be applied directly to the area you are trying to affect. For example, if you are trying to relieve a headache, the temples are the best place to apply as well as across the brow bone and the back of the neck.

If you are someone experiencing thyroid issues, a blend can be formulated and then administered directly on the thyroid. The soles of the feet are another effective area for application, as well as the spine, abdomen, behind the ears, etc.

Neat

Some are best not used neat (without a carrier oil) and must be mixed with another oil which allows the essential oils to sit on top of the skin instead of being directly absorbed so quickly, such as treating eczema or psoriasis or another condition that was best treated topically.

Others, because of certain chemical constituents, actually are irritating to the skin if not mixed with a carrier oil because of the potent properties contained within.

Diffusing

Another way to use essential oils, inhalation of essential oils can be just as beneficial as applying topically. There are many kinds of diffusers, in varying price ranges, the beauty of it is if it seems confusing, it's really not, pick a condition or symptom, you can refer to the Glossary to find out what essential oil best fits the relief you are seeking and it only takes a couple of drops on a diffuser pad or dropped in water (depending on your diffuser) to find the desired relief. So, even if the essential oil was expensive, they last a long time because you typically are only using a couple drops at a time.

Internally With Caution

Some essential oils can be taken internally, again a couple drops in water morning and or night. Some should never be taken internally. Which is why it is important to educate yourself when using them and work with a qualified professional, as with anything.

If you are using prescription meds, you should definitely educate yourself about contraindications, possible side effects, etc., essential oils are no different, in order to be used safely. Some can interact with medications, so it is always best to ask your physician when using prescription medications. And if you are told that they are contraindicated, sometimes, other essential oils can be used instead of others.

Safe

They are so safe that they can be used during pregnancy. Certain ones can be used on babies and children and on our pets, too. If we choose to use essential oils to protect ourselves and our families from prescription medications, our pets are part of our family, too.

Benefits

The benefits of essential oils are so numerous that this reference is not efficient in expressing them.

But a few of the properties include:

- **balancing blood sugar levels**
- **balancing hormone levels**

- increasing circulation
- increase lymphatic drainage
- protecting the internal organs
- supporting a healthy metabolism
- supporting healthy cellular regeneration
- balance sebum production in the skin
- minimize allergy symptoms
- antispasmodic
- anti-inflammatory
- antibacterial
- antifungal
- antiparasitic
- antimicrobial
- lower blood pressure
- lower cholesterol levels
- anticancer
- antidepressant
- anti-tumor
- mood balancing
- fever reducing
- stress relieving
- tension relieving
- dry up mucus
- immune support

Basically, all of the same things that we know herbs do! They are just much more concentrated plant allies and I would probably limit my use of them to topical applications for the beginner.

Do not ever let anyone tell you that you have some condition that nothing can be done for or that you need to take medication for the rest of your life and the symptoms you are experiencing cannot be alleviated. The body is infinite, complex and very basic at the same time; given what it needs, it will function properly, that's it.

If it is deficient, then it just needs to be brought back into balance and then symptoms fall away and start disappearing until overall health is achieved. Not saying it is an overnight occurrence, especially if you are on numerous medications or have numerous conditions, but I can tell you that over time, which will pass anyway (whether you make changes or not,) you will get better, slowly but surely, it will happen and vital health will be achieved. Even if it takes years to reach the goals you desire, either the years will pass and you will strengthen or you will deteriorate, it's up to you.

Summary ~

In this chapter, we learned the way to treat your child, we have a basic understanding of imbalance, the causes and effects of lifestyle choices. We know how to stabilize, detoxify and rebuild after an illness. We understand the Healing Crisis and why it happens, knowing the potential that distilled water has for detoxification and the importance of removing toxic overload so that our immune systems can perform at their optimum level.

Knowing the complexities of herbs and the importance of researching and practicing safety guidelines are now understood. A basis has been laid for the knowledge that because of the cumulative effects of certain herbs, discontinuing use for periods of time during treatment is required.

The Beauty of Herbal Medicine has been explored as well as the vital importance our thoughts play at the time of blending including the value of listening to yourself and any possible plants that pop into your head.

We are now clear as to the dangers of diagnostic tests and the risks involved in a 'routine procedure.' We understand the warnings involved with pharmaceutical medications, including NSAIDS and the effects they have on our joints after 2 years. We know what the leading cause of death is in the US and how to avoid it.

A basis has been laid as to the importance of meeting nutritional requirements to avoid imbalances in both our minds and bodies. We understand how easy it can be to make ourselves feel better and how easy it is to make the right choices and how what is right is not always popular and how what is popular isn't always right.

Grasping the vital importance our emotions have on our health and the connection between what we eat and how we feel is understood. Aware of essential oils and the ways to use them allows us another method of utilizing plant medicine through inhalation and the art of Aromatherapy.

The connection between GMOs, Leaky Gut and Leaky Brain have been made. Understanding how fiber works in the body and the danger inflammation is to our health. We now appreciate the Infinite Intelligence of Mother Nature and value the medicine she has given us.

Chapter 6 ~ Plant Profiles

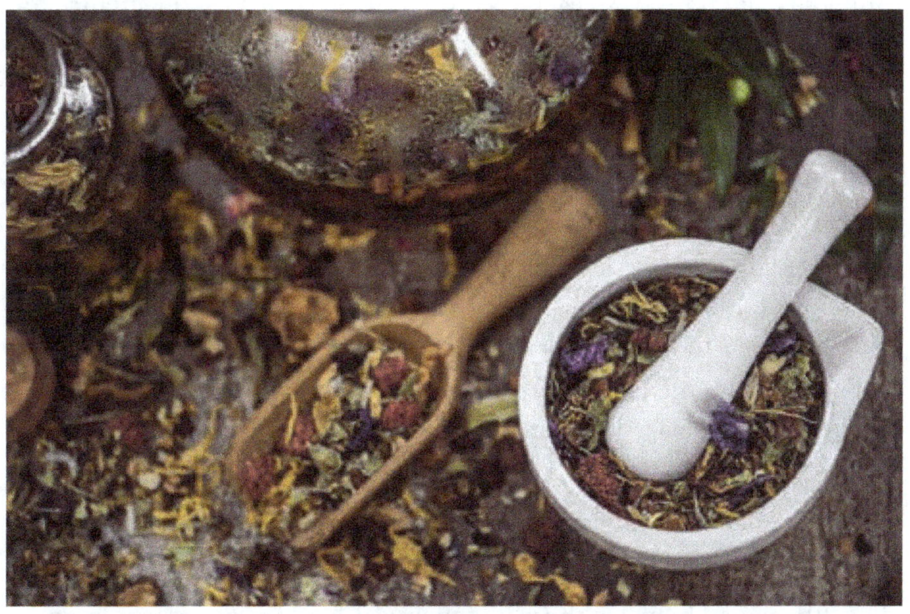

"In all creatures, animals, birds, fishes, herbs and fruit trees mysterious healing powers lie hidden, Which no man can know, unless they are revealed to him by God himself."

– Hildegard von Bingen

Before we explore each Plant Profile, I would like to take a moment to thank all of the dedicated Herbalists who have come before us, who have taken the laborious time of completing the tedious task of recording their experiences with plants. This includes our ancient ancestors literally hand drawing or carving on walls to ensure this sacred knowledge was never lost.

I am honored to bring this information to you passing on the knowledge that I've collected during my time here, exploring the streams and mountains of Vermont, astonished at every turn of the Bounty of Mother

Earth. The diversity of plants she has offered us is so vast that I wonder if Nature's mysteries can ever really be fully discovered.

But with each transcript, each recording of every plant acquaintance, our understanding grows deeper, sinking in the dimensions of our reality, that we all depend on each other, there is an interconnectedness that is both beautiful and as cyclic as the seasons.

Similar to our symbiotic relationship with the trees, giving the air we need to breathe and us supplying them with the adequate air they need.

By providing us with clean air, clean water, clean medicine, clean food if we select it. Nature gives us everything we require to enjoy life, sun, forests, beaches, mountains, deserts with healing plants at our fingertips.

Let's enjoy the medicine she's given us so we can enjoy the life we've been given and share the miracle of health that we are all striving for.

The way herbs work in the body, the course their actions take, is so infinitely seamless that only Divinity could have created such a complex yet simple healing system.

The differences between the phytochemicals and flavonoids, polysaccharides, omega 3s, essential fatty acids, terpenes that each herb holds are similar to its own little prescription specially formulated in Mother Nature's Pharmacy.

Containing specific amounts of each molecule in the perfect formula for relieving so many numbers of symptoms, conditions and ailments that the possible combinations are endless and countless. This is why you should never give up when trying to treat any disease or symptom, once you find the perfect calculations of each specific compound in their adequate quantities developed correctly to your individual specification; then complete healing will resound.

In this chapter, we will explore 7 different Plant Profiles under-standing their uses and applications. We learned preparations in Chapter 4, so each herb does not include preparation instructions, you can refer back for methods of preparing the herbs.

How to Use the Plant Profiles

When studying the plant, notice its curative properties and what conditions it treats and then decide which route of administration you choose. Remember that herbs have a primary function and a secondary function, utilize the primary function for targeting the worst of the symptoms then utilize the secondary functions in a complementary fashion with other herbs that share those actions.

Each herb has its own phytochemical constituents, so if it seems like you're not achieving the desired results within three days or immediately in some cases, mix it up, change the dose, bring in some other allies.

Herbs are recognized like old friends in the body, celebrating their reunion, visiting places they haven't been in a long time, replacing vital compounds, clearing out others, like mini housekeepers, waking up the good guys and kicking the bad guys to the curb, in no uncertain terms.

There are herbs that are known to keep away pathogens that keep coming back, that's their function, is to put an end to it once and for all. To include every constituent found in each herb and its properties is beyond the scope of this book, so I will limit it to descriptions of a few of the active constituents.

If we think of plants as beautiful as they are, like soldiers in our army of natural killers and fighters. They each have their own branches of the military (or of your body) that they target, immune function, respiratory, circulatory, nervous system, sometimes we can go with the milder guys, other times we bring out the Green Berets to divide and conquer.

There's an herb for whatever you seek, whether you're looking for a strong reaction or a mild one, the choice is yours. And the beauty of it, you don't have to spend too much time experimenting because we've done it for you, I have given you recipes and included herbs that have been proven through time, time tested, kid approved to restore balance without suicidal thoughts, brain bleeding, liver failure, thyroid dysfunction, kidney damage, swelling of the face and hands, difficulty breathing, irregular heartbeat, shortness of breath, actually they do the exact opposite, they target all of those symptoms with no side effects. Herbs, controlling the course of an illness can give your body the time needed to restore balance. Come with me on a journey discovering the essence of Plant Medicine…

Patch Test

Some folks show sensitivities to certain species of plants or specific plant types, for sensitive individuals a patch test can be performed prior to treatment to determine if there are any sensitivities.

Method for Essential Oils

Dilute one drop of essential oil in four drops of carrier oil. Apply dime-sized amount of this blend to a small area of skin that is not sensitive.

Wait a few hours and see if skin reacts.

Do not use near eyes and or nose, ears or any other particularly sensitive areas of skin.

Salve or Oil Method

Apply a small amount to skin and wait a few hours to see if there's any reaction. Most herbs are so gentle, there's nothing to worry about, for those who have sensitivities, better to be safe than sorry.

Arnica

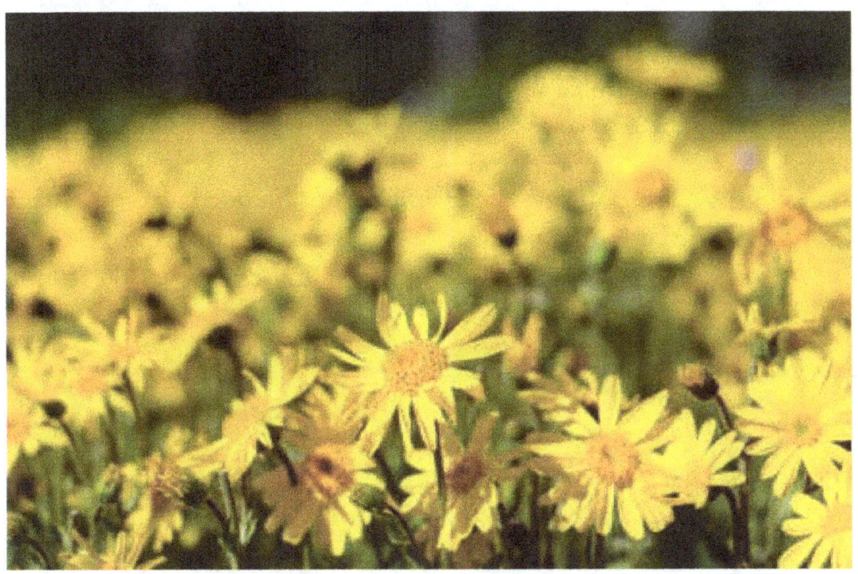

"If spots and blisters erupt between the skin and flesh, then let the person cook the herb in water and wrap the blemishes, and then the person will be healed."

— *Hildegard of Bingen*

Arnica - *Arnica Montana, Arnica Helvetica* G.Don ex Loudon

Other names: Leopard's Bane, Wolfsbane, Mountain Tobacco, Mountain Arnica

Genus of perennial, herbaceous plants in the Asteraceae plant family also called *Compositae*

Native to the mountains of Europe and Siberia also found in mountainous areas of Canada, the northern US and Europe

Name Origin: Thought to have been derived from the Greek word, 'arni,' which means lamb, after its soft hairy leaves.

Notes:

Goethe brewed Arnica tea aiding in his recovery from a heart attack, extending his life and speeding his recovery.

Used since the sixteenth century.

Part used: flower

Curative Properties: analgesic, anesthetic, antihemorrhagic, anticoagulant, anti-inflammatory, antiphlogistic, antiviral, diaphoretic, diuretic, emollient, expectorant, hemostatic, immunostimulant, pectoral, stimulant, vasodilators, vulnerary

Energy and flavor: warm, poisonous

Cautions:

1. DO NOT APPLY DIRECTLY TO SKIN: Use in oil form or Homeopathic Remedy, essential oil is not recommended for inhalation, because of its strong potency.

2. Never use directly on broken or damaged skin.

3. If you have allergies to the *Asteraceae* or *Compositae* family including ragweed, chrysanthemums, marigolds, daisies, possible sensitivities can occur. Perform a patch test first, if needed.

4. Pregnant and breastfeeding women should refrain from using Arnica oil.

Conditions: arthritis, broken bones, bruising, carpal tunnel, contusions, hair loss, hematomas, muscle aches, muscle tenderness, osteoarthritis, rheumatic diseases, sprains, subcutaneous blood capillaries, wounds

Biochemical constituents: alkaloids, amines, carbohydrates, coumarins, flavonoids (e.g., eupafolin, patuletin, spinacetin), terpenoids (e.g., arnifolin, arnicolides, helenalin), volatile oils (e.g., thymol, ethers of thymol), thymol, potent anti-inflammatory helenalin, a sesquiterpene lactone, phenolic acids, resins, bitters (arnicin), tannins and carotenoids

Note: Properties of flavonoids show antioxidative properties helping to prevent heart disease, cancer and immunodeficiency viruses. Protecting the inner wall of the vessel, flavonoids help prevent plaque buildup in the arteries and narrowing of vessel walls.

Parts of the body: blood, circulation

Preparations~

Poultice:
Use tea made from the flowers for a compress on the stomach to relieve abdominal pain.

Doctors have used it for internal bleeding and as a cardiac agent.

External wash:
1 heaping tsp. flowers
1 cup water

Steep
Use cold on wounds, not on broken or open skin, mostly for bruising and swelling.

Oil Infusion Preparation:
1 oz. flowers
1 oz. Olive oil
Heat flowers in Olive oil in a water bath, such as a double boiler for a few hours.
Strain through several layers of cheesecloth
Cap, label
Apply directly onto affected area two to four times a day
Massage into scalp for hair loss

Homeopathic Dose:

1 to 4 pellets under the tongue

Can be administered every 15 minutes for trauma.

Use either 30c or 30x, 6c or 6x -

Give 1 to 4 pellets under the tongue depending on the severity of the injury.

<u>More Information</u>: Arnica oil is an excellent topical remedy, applied directly to injury as long as there is no broken or damaged skin. This is one herb I definitely recommend having in your First Aid Kit in its Homeopathic form, gentle enough to not have to worry about but effective enough to not want to be caught without it.

Whether it is a bump or a bruise, broken bone, sprain, etc. it is an excellent anti-inflammatory herb. If I didn't have Arnica with me, the duration of pain and emotional trauma compared to times when I had it and times when I did not were not even comparable. Its benefits are so effective. Gentle enough to give to toddlers who are always falling down. Suggested dose above.

Calendula

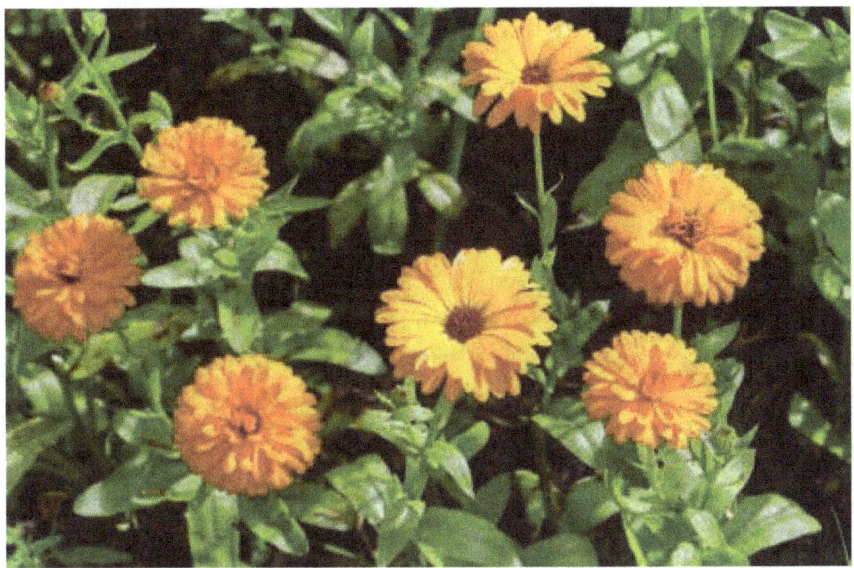

"Calendula strengthens the heart exceedingly."

— Nicolas Culpeper

Calendula - *Calendula Officinalis*

Other names: Scotch Marigold, Pot Marigold, Common Marigold, Ruddles

Genus: herbaceous flowering annual in the Asteraceae family

Native to Western Europe, Southeastern Asia, the Mediterranean

Name Origin: noted for its habit of blooming on the first day of the month, according to the ancient Julian calendar.

Notes:

Being considered sacred in India, using the flowers to adorn statues and deities. In the twelfth century in Macers Herbal, it is recommended that by simply looking at it will improve eyesight, clear the head, and encourage cheerfulness. They were used in religious ceremonies in ancient Aztec and Mayan civilizations. In Germany, it is used in soups and stews, as well as a saffron substitute.

Parts used: flowers

Curative Properties: antibiotic, anticancer, antidiarrhetic, antifungal, antihemorrhagic, antiinflammatory, antimicrobial, antiphlogistic, antipyretic, antispasmodic, antiseptic, antiviral, aperient, astringent, cholagogue, decongestant, demulcent, detergent, diaphoretic, emmenagogue, emollient, febrifuge, hemostatic, immunomodulator, lymphatic, muscle relaxant, mucilaginous, stimulant, stimulates bile production, vulnerary, wound healing

Energy and flavors: neutral, bitter, spicy

Cautions:

1. Not to be taken internally during pregnancy or breast-feeding or even those seeking to get pregnant should avoid, as it can potentially cause miscarriage due to the highly potent pro- menstruation effects.

2. Those with allergies to plants in the Asteraceae/Compositae family might show sensitivities. Other plants in this family include Ragweed, Chamomile and Echinacea.

3. Possible interactions with sedatives due to its muscle relaxing abilities, as well as diabetes and blood pressure medications.

Conditions: abscesses, boils, bruises, burns, cancer, colitis, constipation, cradle cap, diaper rash, diarrhea, earaches, fevers, headaches, gingivitis and gum disease, hot flashes, infection, injuries, eruptive skin diseases (such as measles, shingles, thrush), lymphatic issues, menstrual cramps, mouth ulcers, pain from injuries and irritation, promotes healing, pulled muscles, pus formation, shingles, sores, sprains, stops bleeding, stomach cramps, swollen glands, ulcers, vomiting, warts

Biochemical constituents: organic iodine which accounts for its antiseptic qualities, calendic and linoleic acid fatty acids, flavonoids, carotenoids, lutein and beta-carotene, monoterpenes and sesquiterpenes

Parts of the body: heart, liver, lungs, reproductive system, skin, stomach

Preparations~

Tincture:
3- 10 drops

Tea:
1 tsp.
1.1/2 cup almost boiling water

Water Infusion:
1 to 2 tsp. flowers 1 cup of water
Steep

Dose:
Take 1/2 tbs. every hour

Oil Infusion:
8 ounces of flowers
16 oz. of extra virgin olive oil
In mason jar, cover flowers with oil

Shake everyday infusing with healing intention for 3-6 weeks depending on how strong of an infusion you want
Strain, cap, label.

Mouthwash:
Use tea

Juice:
For warts, rub directly on wart.

Ulcers Relief Tea:
Equal parts
Calendula
Marshmallow root
Valerian
Cramp bark
Pint hot water

Earache:
Put 2 drops on cotton ball and hold in ear.

<u>More Information</u>: This is another herb in our *Cancer-Free Protocol*. When I inquired of the Herbalist at the farmers' market in the very beginning, Calendula was one of the main herbs in her herbal blend that I began giving my husband. I continued to give him this tea blend all throughout treatment. My Immunity Tea blend also has Calendula in it.

Calendula is another one of my favorite flowers to grow, the flowers have so many variations in tone and color from one seed pack, ranging from creamy yellow to dark orange to creamy yellow on the top of the petals and deep orange on the bottom! So easy, from growing and saving the seeds to making the healing oil extracting the medicinal benefits offered.

A truly wonderful plant for children to enjoy, from graciously picking the flowers for salads to pouring the golden oil over them in the jar and shaking every day charging them with loving energy. The oil is excellent for any kind of skin condition.

I use it in my Healing Salve and I've received over 50 testimonials for alleviating the discomfort associated with eczema and psoriasis from those suffering from those symptoms, who had tried everything before with no success.

Chamomile

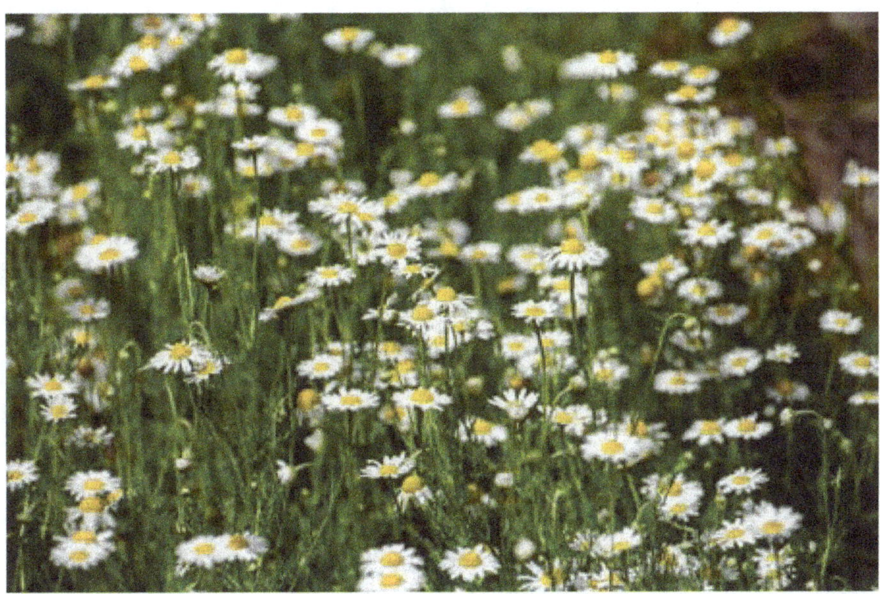

"Peter was not very well during the evening. His mother put him to bed, and made some chamomile tea: One table-spoonful to be taken at bedtime."

— *Beatrix Potter*

Chamomile - German *Chamomilla Recutita*, Roman

Chamaemelum Nobile

Other names: Hungarian Chamomile, Pineapple Weed. Saxon word for *Chamomile* is *Maythen*

New England's wild variety is known as Pineapple Weed.

Sometimes referred to as Herbal Aspirin.

Genus: members of the Asteraceae/Compositae family,

German Chamomile is an anuual

Roman Chamomile is a perennial

Native to Western Europe and Northern Africa

Name Origin: Greek, '*khamai*,' meaning 'on the ground,' and melon, meaning 'apple.'

Notes:

Roman variety flower heads are larger.

German Chamomile is taller than the Roman variety.

German Chamomile possesses greater anti-inflammatory properties.

All varieties generally have the same medicinal properties.

Has been used for nearly 5,000 years.

Known by the Anglo-Saxons as Maythen, one of nine sacred herbs given to the World by the God, Woden.

Known as the Plant's Physician because it's thought to cure whatever ailments the plant near it is suffering from. Makes a great companion plant in the garden, ensuring the health of other surrounding plants.

Egyptian noblewomen were said to have crushed Chamomile flowers and applied them to their skin preserving their youthful glow and naturally slowing the signs of aging.

Has been approved in 26 countries to treat colic, indigestion, muscle spasms, tension, inflammation, infection.

One cup of Chamomile tea has two calories, two milligrams of sodium and no cholesterol.

Parts used: flowers

Curative Properties: alterative, analgesic, anesthetic, anodyne, antacid, antibiotic, anticancer, anticoagulant, antidepressant, antidiarrhetic, antihistamine, anti-inflammatory, antiseptic, antispasmodic, calmative, carminative, decongestant, deodorant, diaphoretic, diuretic, febrifuge nervine, orexigenic, parasiticide, restorative, sedative, stimulant, stomachic, tonic, vermifuge

Energy and flavors: neutral, aromatic, bitter, spicy

Cautions:

1. Hormone-sensitive conditions, such as endometriosis, fibroids, or cancers of the breast, uterus and ovaries should avoid using Chamomile because it may act like estrogen in the body.

2. Chamomile is a mild uterine stimulant so if you're pregnant, speak with a midwife before ingesting Chamomile extracts (mild Chamomile tea shouldn't cause any problems).

Conditions: acid reflux, allergies (seasonal), anxiety, arthritis, asthma, bruises, burns, cancer, canker sores, childhood digestive issues, colds, colic, conjunctivitis, constipation, dandruff, dark spots, depression, diarrhea (seasonal), digestive complaints, eczema, edema, fatigue, fevers, fine lines, flu, gingivitis, gout, hemorrhoids, hysteria, indigestion, inflammatory, insomnia, irritable bowel syndrome, jaundice, menstrual cramps, migraines, motion sickness, muscle soreness, muscle spasms, nausea, nervous diseases, nervousness, neuralgia, nightmares, oligomenorrhea, open sores, pain, PMS, sciatica, sinus infection, slipped disc, stress, sties, swelling, teething, toothaches, upset stomach, vomiting (prevent), whooping cough, worms, wounds

Biochemical constituents: anodyne compounds, chamazulene, easily assimilated calcium content, flavonoids, including apigenin, quercetin, patuletin, coumarin, glucosides, heterosides, tannic acid, terpenoids

Parts of the body: hair, kidneys, liver, lungs, reproductive organs, spleen, stomach

Preparations~

Capsules Dose:
73 to 366 milligrams per day, for about 8 weeks

Tea:
One to two times per day

Colic Tea:
1 tsp. flowers
2 cups of water
May be given to babies

Variations:
Blend with Lemon Balm, Peppermint, Anise, Fennel, Caraway

For a less bitter infusion, steep shorter amount of time, the longer it steeps the more bitter it will be.

Relaxing Bath Infusion:
Or for relieving skin issues:
1 tbs. flowers
1 cup water
Pour in bath, soak

Variations:
Add Roses, Lavender, Calendula flowers

Pain Relieving Infusion:
1/2 oz. flowers
Pint of water

Dose:
Drink 1/2 cup at a time -

In a study of people taking pain medication, 10 out of 12 people who drank Chamomile tea instead of taking their pain medication at bedtime fell into a deep restful sleep within 10 minutes.

Gargle:
For mouth and throat inflammation

Hair Rinse:
3 tbs. flowers
1 cup water
Rinse hair after conditioner, restores natural color giving it a healthy sheen

Sore Eye Wash Tea:
1 tbs. flowers
1 ½ cup water
Wash eye as needed

Astral Travel Dream Pillow
Equal parts
Mugwort
Lavender
Roses
Chamomile
1 part Rosemary
1 part Orris root
Blend in a glass or stainless steel bowl.
Spoon (never use plastic) in a little pouch
Place under your pillow or inside your pillowcase

<u>More Information</u>: If you have children in the house, this will be one of your go to herbs! See the list of symptoms it treats? Everything, right?

Easy to grow and another one that can be enjoyed in salads, sweet-smelling, if you plant it near your walkway, every time you brush by, it will give off a whiff of sweet-smelling goodness. Friends with everyone in the garden, it gets along with everyone, so you can plant it anywhere.

A cup of tea makes a great nighttime ritual to wind the kiddos down after a big day, as they sink into a good book. If you could only have one herb in your garden, this one might be a good candidate!

Echinacea

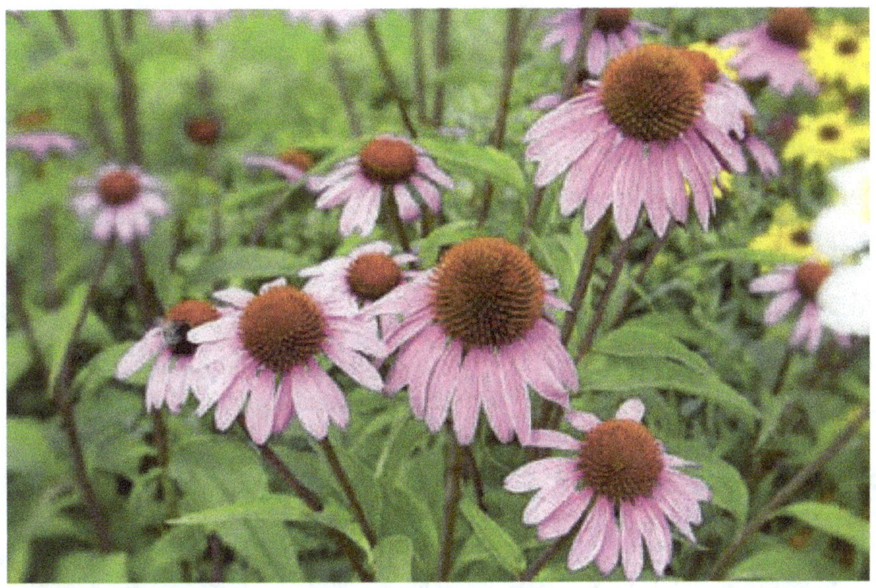

"Its extraordinary powers—anti fermentative and antizymotic—are well shown in its power over changes produced in the fluids of the body, whether from internal causes or from aexternal introductions. As a stimulant to the capillary circulation, no remedy is comparable with it, and it endows the vessels with a recuperative power or formative force, so as to enable them to successfully resist local inflammatory processes due to debility and blood depravation."

— Harvey Wickes Felter Eclectic Physician

Echinacea *- Echinacea Purpurea, Echinacea Angustifolia*

In Cancer-Free Protocol

Other names: Snake Root, Coneflower, Prairie, Purple Coneflower, Sampson Root, Black Sampson, Red Sunflower

Genus: Perennial, Asteraceae family

Native to Midwest, North American

Name Origin: Echinacea derives from the Greek, 'echinos' (hedgehog) and refers to the thorny base of the flower head.

Purpurea is Latin for 'purple-red.'

Notes:

Used for 400 years by the Great Plains Indian tribes.

Been known as the Great Herbal Diplomat.

Used for treatment with the early settlers.

Native American remedy for snakebites.

Eclectic medicine was founded around the 1850s by Dr. Wooster Beach, a specialist in the integration of Native American herbs and Homeopathic medicine and the scientific knowledge of the day. Echinacea was part of this herbal medicine movement bringing in thousands of highly qualified and dedicated doctors. Throughout the country, they sold these Eclectic medicines. Their system of diagnosis resembled the thousands of year old medical systems that evolved in China and India, including but not limited to evaluations of the tongue and pulse. Their main college was in Cincinnati Ohio and by the late 1930s, it was closed.

Not having grasped the concepts of blending multiple herbs together to create complex formulations utilizing different plant components as their predecessors in China and India had. The Eclectic's popularized the use of Echinacea root to treat inflammation. With the onset of the discovery of penicillin, Echinacea was soon forgotten, unfortunately. With the increase of synthetic medicines, the Eclectic's influence faded. The Lloyd Library in Cincinnati is probably the greatest herbal medical library in the world. It contains all of the accumulated herbal knowledge of the Eclectic's including a current catalog of books and journals on herbal medicine that was published and enjoyed worldwide.

Parts used: flowers, root, leaves

Curative Properties: adaptogen, alterative, anesthetic, antibacterial, antibiotic, anticancer, anticatarrhal, antifungal, antiinflammatory, anti-microbial, antipyretic, antiseptic, anti venomous, antiviral, blood cleanser, bronchodilatory, cleanser, carminative, decongestant, demulcent, diaphoretic, diuretic, febrifuge, immunostimulant, laxative, lymphatic tonic, maturating, parasiticide, purgative, sialagogue, stimulant, tonic

Energy and flavors: cool, bitter, pungent

Cautions: take treatment for 2 weeks on, 2 weeks off, then start again if needed.

Conditions: AIDS, anxiety, arthritic diseases, asthma, bacterial infections (acute), bloodstream infections, boils, cancer, colds, constipation, croup, depression, diphtheria, fevers, flu, food poisoning, gangrene, genital herpes, gonorrhea, gum disease, influenza, inflammation, kidney infection, malaria, migraines, pain, poison oak, poison ivy, respiratory tract infections (upper), rheumatoid arthritis, septicemia, sinusitis (acute), skin eruptions, slow-healing wounds, snake bites, social phobias, sore throat, strep throat, syphilis, tonsillitis, toothache, tuberculosis, typhoid, urinary tract infection, vaginal yeast infections, venomous bites, viral infections, whooping cough

Biochemical constituents: flavonoids, inulin, polysaccharides, phytochemicals, vitamin C

Parts of the body: immune system, liver, lungs, stomach

Preparations~

Tea:

1 tsp. of root, leaves

2 cups of water

(flowers are usually big, you would need to put 1 to a pint of water)

Dose:

½ cup of tea can be taken every 3 hours
Doses can be tapered down to 2 times a day for a week or two until symptoms have disappeared.

Tincture:

I dropper

2 oz warer

Usually my preferred route of administration

Use either or all: roots, flowers, leaves

Dose:

Take 1 to 3 ml dose every 2 to 3 hours

5 to 15 drops for lighter dose

Tea or tincture can be taken every 2 hours in small frequent doses

Decoction Dose:

Take 5 ml every 3 hours

Capsules Dose:

1 g of dried powder

Follow directions on the bottle or make your own with a dried, ground plant.

Sore Throat Gargle:

20 drops tincture

½ cup water

1 ounce of decoction

Immune Stimulation:

Dose:

5 mg of Echinacea per one kilogram of body weight taken daily over 10 days period is effective as an immune system stimulant, studies have shown.

The medical journal *Hindawi* published material suggesting that Echinacea stops viral colds, nothing they're going to find if they test OTC cold medicines.

Echinacea cuts the chances of catching a common cold by 58 percent, reducing the duration of the common cold by almost one-and-a-half days, according to a study conducted by the University of Connecticut.

Anxiety, Depression, Social Phobia Relief Dose:

Take 5mg mg at a time - and no more!

In fact, it's thought that taking more than 20 milligrams per dose can actually cancel out the Echinacea benefits that relieve anxiety.

<u>More Information</u>: I have been familiar with this herb for over 20 years, my first line of defense when my girls started showing any signs of illness. Little runny nose, cough, through experience, I learned of its efficacy. My girls hardly ever got really sick, they'd come down with a cold, but soon enough it was gone and it never lingered or turned into something worse. Echinacea was one of my first friends who introduced me to the healing benefits of plants and spurred my curiosity to see what else plants could combat or conquer.

With its natural antibiotic qualities, it raises the body's natural resistance to infection by stimulating and aiding the immune system. By increasing macrophages and T cell activity, which are white blood cells that protect against invasion by viruses and bacteria.

Elder

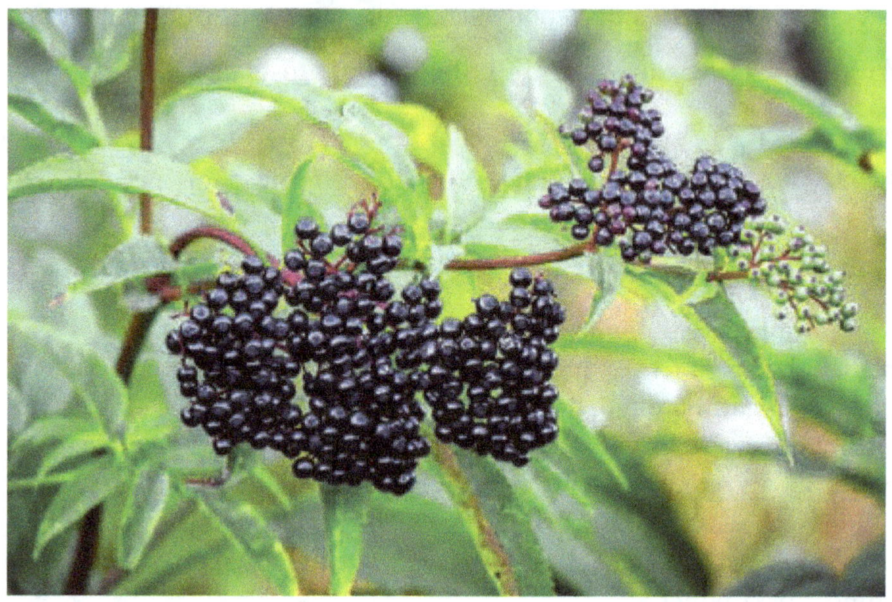

"The Russians believe that Elder-trees drive away evil spirits, and the Bohemians go to it with a spell to take away fever. The Sicilians think that sticks of its wood will kill serpents and drive away robbers, and the Serbs introduce a stick of Elder into their wedding ceremonies to bring good luck. In England it was thought that the Elder was never struck by lightning, and a twig of it tied into three or four knots and carried in the pocket was a charm against rheumatism. A cross made of Elder and fastened to cowhouses and stables was supposed to keep all evil from the animals."

— Lady Northcote

Elder - *Sambucus Nigra*

Other names: Black Elder, European Elder, European Elderberry, European Black Elderberry

Genus: flowering plants in the family Adoxaceae

Native to Europe, Africa, parts of Asia, more and more common in the U.S

Name Origin: From the Anglo-Saxon word 'aeld,' it was called 'Eldrun' in Anglo-Saxon Days, which becomes 'Hyldor' and 'Hyllantree' in the fourteenth century. Appearing as 'Ellhorn' in low Saxon.

Notes:

Evidence gives reason to believe that Elderberries were cultivated by pre-historic man.

Known to the Egyptians.

Listed by Hippocrates in his Materia Medica.

Described as a complete medicine chest.

Spoke of as a blood purifier by Pliny and Culpeper.

Recipes for Elderberry-based medications going back to Ancient Egypt.

Used to promote labor and childbirth by some Indians using root and bark tea.

Should be planted near the house because it cannot be struck by lightning, according to Folklore.

Thought to protect those in the house from evil spirits and disease.

Thought of as a charm to give health and good luck, a twig was carried close to the body.

Prescribed juice for neuralgia and sciatica in Europe.

Attracts more than 35 different birds!

Parts used: bark, berries, flowers, leaves

Bark: blood purifier, constipation, diuretic, emetic, emollient, liver stimulant, purgative

Berries: blood purifier

Flowers: antihistamine, discutient, exanthematous, gentle stimulant, mild astringent, rubefacient

Leaves: bruises, skin irritations, sprains

Curative Properties: alterative, anticatarrhal, antidiarrhetic, antihistamine, antiinflammatory, antioxidant, antipyretic, antirheumatic, antiviral, circulatory stimulant, diaphoretic, diuretic, emetic, expectorant, febrifuge, hepatic, immunomodulator, immunostimulant, laxative, pectoral, promotes sweating, purgative

Energy and flavors: cool, hot, acrid, bitter, dry

Cautions:

1. Only the Black Elder is safe to use internally. Red Elder is toxic.

2. Do not eat raw uncooked berries in any great quantity as they can cause digestive upset and diarrhea.

3. Fresh plants can cause poisoning, children have been poisoned by chewing or sucking on the bark. Cooked berries are safe.

4. Autoimmune disease sufferers, such as rheumatoid arthritis, should ask their Healthcare Provider before taking Elderberry because it may stimulate the immune system.

5. People with organ transplants should not take Elderberry.

6. Possible interactions with medication because of its strong medicinal benefits.

Note: If taking any of these, consult your Healthcare Provider before using:

- diabetes medications

- diuretics (water pills)

- chemotherapy

- immunosuppressants (including corticosteroids (prednisone) and medications used to treat autoimmune diseases)

- laxatives

- Theophylline (TheoDur)

Conditions: bronchitis, colds, epilepsy, eruptive diseases, fevers, flu, headaches, herpes, influenza, measles, mouth ulcers, rash, rheumatism, shingles, sore throat, tonsillitis, upper respiratory infection, viruses

Berries: arthritic, diarrhea, rheumatic complaints

Flowers: burns, rashes, minor skin ailments, wrinkles, twitching eyelids, bronchitis

Leaves: detoxifying agent

Biochemical constituents:

- **Bark**: viburnum acid, tannic acid, chlorophyll, grape sugar, gum, starch, pectin, fat, wax, alkaline and earthy salts

- **Fruit**: high in vitamin C, quercetin, kaempferol, rutin, and phenolic acids, flavonoids, anthocyanidins, vitamin A, vitamin B6, iron and potassium

- **Leaf**: alkaloid, a purgative resin, glycoside

- **Flowers**: semi-solid volatile oil

- **European flowers**: 0.3 percent of an essential oil composed of free fatty acids and alkanes. The triterpenes alpha- and betaamyrin, ursolic acid, oleanolic acid, betulin, betulinic acid

- **Berries**: rich in vitamins A and C

Parts of the body: kidneys, liver, lungs, mouth

Preparations~

Infusion:

1 tsp.
2 cups water

Tincture:

Take 10 to 20 drops two or three times a day.

Eye Wash:

Use infusion for inflamed or sore eyes.

Elderberry Syrup

When using fresh berries, use twice the amount of dried berries that your
recipe recommends.

Ingredients:

1 cup dried Elderberries
Possible additions - Wild Cherry Bark, Licorice, Mullein, Echinacea
4 cups of water
1 cup raw local honey or organic maple syrup
(double the amount of sweetener to increase shelf life)
1 cup organic grain alcohol (vodka or brandy)

This is recommended for extending shelf life, but you could keep it in
the fridge as an alternative, too, if it's for children.

Directions:

Combine berries and herbs with cold water in a pot and bring to a simmer.

Reduce heat and allow herbs to simmer for 30 to 40 minutes.

Remove from heat and let steep for 1 hour.

Strain berries and herbs using a funnel overlaid with doubled cheesecloth or undyed cotton muslin bag and squeeze out liquid (careful, liquid will likely still be hot!).

Discard used herbs in compost.

Once liquid has cooled to just above room temperature:

Add honey and stir, warming not above 110 degrees so as to not kill beneficial enzymes in honey.

Store in sterilized bottles, label.

Will keep in fridge for several weeks.

Freckle Removing Infusion: (there's nothing wrong with freckles)
1 tsp. herbs
1 cup water
Soak flowers in water overnight.
Strain and use as wash several times a day.

Influenza Tea:
Blend flowers with Peppermint tea
Drink a cup every few hours.

Gargle/Mouthwash for Mouth Ulcers, Sore Throat, Tonsillitis:
Use tea

Recipe~
Elderberry Flower Fritters
Dip in egg and breading and deep fry

Try breading Dandelion flowers too for a Flower Fritter Party!

More Information: Elder and I go way back, utilizing the potent benefits it contains for coughs and lung disorders, this is a #1 'go-to' herb for any household with children. The Elderberry syrup's properties are so much more than just cough syrup. Any cold or cough treated with Elder will soon see relief! And the cough syrup is fun and easy to make.

This is a much better remedy to give your child when they don't feel good as opposed to any OTC medications that actually decrease their immune function and tax their kidneys and liver. This is one remedy that you can feel good about giving to your family because it is good for everyone!

Hemp

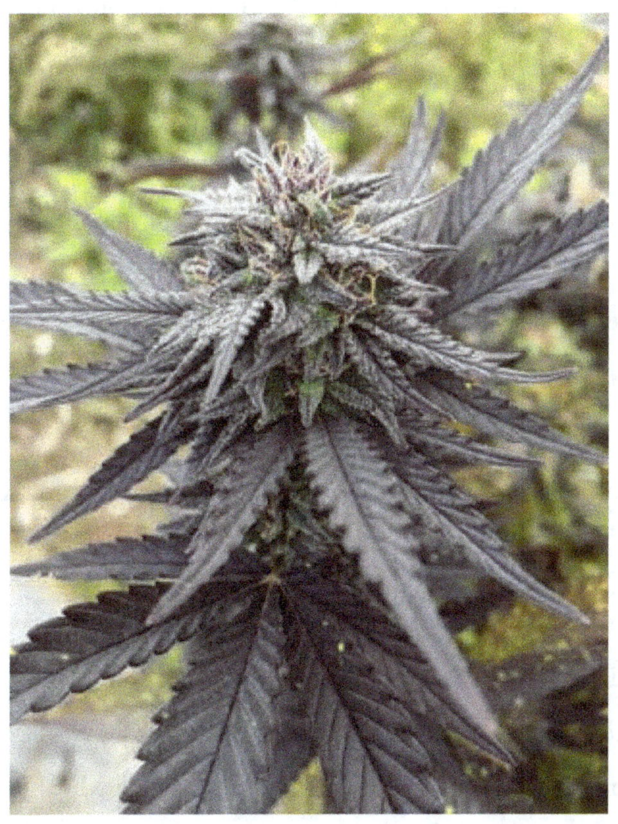

'"Hemp: the only plant that can feed you, house you, clothe you, and heal you."

- Unknown

Hemp - Cannabis Sativa, Cannabis Indica,Cannabis Ruderalis, Da Ma (Chinese) Hou Ma Ren

Other names: Marijuana, Ganja, Grass, Reefer, Mary Jane, Herb, Weed

Genus: Cannabis in the Cannabaceae family, annual, flowering dioecious herb

Native to Asia

Name Origin: The strains of Cannabis are actually 3000-Year-Old Salskrit terms – Sativa 'for daytime,' Indica 'for nighttime.'

Notes:

Cannabis Sativa evolved over 34 million years ago.

Cannabinoid receptors are 600 million years old.

Ma Gu, the Chinese goddess, whose name literally means 'Hemp Maiden,' is associated with longevity and the elixir of life.

The Chinese term that is used for anesthesia is composed with the Chinese character that means 'hemp.'

Hua Tuo, a Han Dynasty physician, is renowned for being the first person to use Cannabis as an anesthetic, for use both internally and externally, by mixing the dried and powdered plant with wine. He was able to perform surgeries controlling the pain of his patients with this preparation (known as Ma Fei San) in conjunction with acupuncture.

One of the most powerful, unique, healing substances on Earth.

Used for 10,000 years.

Chinese described Cannabis in 2000 BCE

Unique among thousands of plants people have used.

CBD stands for Cannabidiol which is a cannabinoid.

Cannabidiol is an anti-psychoactive component and balances out the effects of THC.

THC stands for Delta 9-tetrahydrocannabinol and is the psychoactive component in the plant. It is another cannabinoid found in the plant.

In Physica, Hildegard described using Cannabis seeds therapeutically in great detail, according to Robert Clark and Mark Merlin authors of Cannabis; Evolution and Ethnobotany:

'Hemp (Harif) is hot, and it grows where the air is neither very hot nor very cold, and its nature is similar. Its seed is salubrious, and good as food for healthy people. It is gentle and profitable to the stomach, taking away a bit of its mucus. It is easy to digest, diminishes bad humor's and fortifies good humor's. Nevertheless if one who is weak in the head, and as a vacant brain eats Hemp, it easily afflicts his head. It does not harm one who has a healthy head and full brain. In one who is very ill it even afflicts his stomach a bit. Eating it does not harm one who is moderately ill. Let one who has cold stomach cook Hemp in water and, when the water has been squeezed out, wrap it in a small cloth, and frequently place it, warm on his stomach. This strengthens and renews that area. Also, a cloth made from Hemp is good for binding ulcers and wounds since the heat it has been tempered.'

(Translation by Throop 1998, following the Schott edition based on the 1533 original Physica.)

Colonies in Virginia used it to pay their taxes in 1683-1700 and used to be required to grow it.

One of the first Model Ts ran on Hemp fuel.

The Declaration of Independence was drafted on Hemp paper.

Found in 1920 pharmacopoeia for pain relief and for sleep.

When the DEA started the prohibition, they made up the word, 'Marijuana,' to pass the Marijuana Tax Act of 1937, making it illegal. They used the most common Mexican girl name, 'Mary' and they used the most common Mexican boy name, 'Juan' and put them together to make 'Marijuana.'

Dr. Woodward of the American Medical Association is on record saying that they (the MDs) would have tried to protest that law from passing if they had known it was Cannabis because they were aware of the benefits. Making Cannabis illegal removed a valuable tool from their medicine belt.

Prior to 1937, Cannabis tinctures were available over-the-counter.

Doctors used it as an integral part of the pharmacopeia.

By 1942, Cannabis was out of the American Pharmacopeia, lost all of its connection to medicine and was a dangerous drug.

CBD oil is an extract, not a tincture, tinctures contain alcohol.

CBD oil is Hemp oil extracted in one of any number of ways into either Coconut oil, Hempseed oil, Olive oil, MCT Coconut oil, etc.

Parts used: buds, leaves, seeds

Curative Properties: analgesic, anticancer, antidiabetic, antiemetic, anti-hypertensive, antiinflammatory, antimetastatic, antioxidant, antiproliferative, antispasmodic, antitumor, emollient, expectorant, immune modulator, immunostimulant, maintains homeostasis, nervine, sedative

Energy and flavors: cooling, neutral, sweet

Cautions: none

Conditions: Alzheimer's, arthritis, autoimmune disease, cancer, Crohn's disease, Huntington's, IBS, inflammation, insomnia, Lyme disease, migraines, muscular dystrophy, pain, Parkinson's, plantar fasciitis, rheumatoid arthritis, rheumatism, scoliosis

Biochemical constituents: vitamins A, C, E naturally occurring, B complex, minerals like zinc, potassium calcium, iron magnesium, terpenes, chlorophyll, plant waxes, contains all 20 amino acids

Body Parts: whole body

Preparations~

People do extract Hemp with alcohol as well as other solvents such as butane and propane that I would never recommend. While CO_2 is the preferred extraction method, old style alcohol extraction can be effective as well.

Because of the potential loss of vital compounds, I would recommend acquiring an oil that is a CO_2 extraction. This doesn't mean that you can't grow your own, just that you would give the raw product to a lab-tested facility to process it for you.

Preparation:
Tincture:
Fill jar halfway with fresh or dried herb
Cover with organic grain alcohol
Cap, label, shake everyday infusing with healing intention, love and gratitude
After 1 month strain

Oil Infusion:
Fill jar halfway with fresh or dried herb
Cover with carrier oil (extra virgin olive, safflower, hempseed)
Label, shake every day infusing with healing intention, love and gratitude
After 1 month strain.

Sore Muscle Rub:
Blend in an amber bottle:
1 part Arnica oil
1 part Hemp oil (if Co2 extract, use between 100-200mg)
1 part Hempseed Oil
Essential Oils-
5 drops Frankincense
5 drops Myrrh
5 drops Lemongrass
Apply to affected area topically as needed

Medical Condition Research

Cannabis and Hemp, in essence, are both the same plant, Hemp has a much lower THC content, but both possess cannabinoids.

Hemp plant contains over 500 different compounds, over 120 different cannabinoids and over 200 different terpenes.

Some of the 120 cannabinoids include but are not limited to CBD, THC, CBG, CBC and CBN. This illustration gives a brief description of a number of the cannabinoids that have been researched more extensively. This sacred plant is a strong antioxidant.

Of the 120 cannabinoids present, Cannabidiol and THC are the two that have been researched the most. In that research, they have found over 250 medical conditions that they treat. Now they are beginning to research CBN, CBG and others and the results are astounding!

Over a hundred articles on PubMed have been written about our Endocannabinoid System, this is a well-established understanding of both human and animal physiology.

Endocannabinoid Deficiencies

The following conditions are a symptom of an Endocannabinoid deficiency. Of these conditions cannabinoids have proven beneficial for include but are not limited to:

- Alzheimer's
- Parkinson's
- Seizure disorders
- Anxiety
- neurological disorders
- AIDs
- HIV
- Migraines
- PMS
- IBS
- Autoimmune diseases such as:
    1. fibromyalgia
    2. lupus, etc.

Sea Squirts have a CB receptor almost identical to the human CB1 receptor.

If you do a PubMed search and look for the number of peer-reviewed scientific articles that describe the Endocannabinoid System, there has been an average of one article published every other day for the last 20 years.

Endocannabinoid System

Our bodies have an Endocannabinoid System that was discovered over 20 years ago. Similar to our Endocrine System, with CB1 and CB2 receptors all throughout our body regulating just about every physiological system in our bodies ranging from pain relief to insomnia, anxiety, regulating sebum (oil) production in our skin, etc.

This is a lock and key system, CBDs bind to those receptors, turns out we are hardwired by Mother Nature to receive the benefits of this plant! It triggers healing in our bodies.

Our Endocannabinoid System is an integrative system of homeostasis, with CBDs causing the release and balance of our internal cannabinoids. Hemp produces phytocannabinoids. Our bodies produce endocannabinoids, not as much as we would like, this is why when we use CBD it feels so good because it resonates with our bodies on a cellular level.

This is a real physiological system discovered over 20 years ago, in 1988 by Dr. Allyn Howlett. CB1 and CB2 Receptors are very similar. The primary function of the Endocannabinoid System is cellular homeostasis as we've said.

Manipulation of the Endocannabinoid System may provide effective treatment for a wide variety of diseases. It down regulates inflammation. These are receptors in our body that have been hardwired over eons of time to access these compounds and utilize them to balance out our systems.

Stimulates regeneration of brain tissue.

CB1 and CB2 Receptors

CB1 and CB2 receptors are found all throughout the body.

• **CB1 Receptors:** Central nervous system, testes, uterus, reproductive

tissues, adipose tissue, connective tissue, endocrine glands, leukocytes, spleen, heart, GI tract, liver, organs
• **CB2 Receptors:** immune system, monocytes, macrophages, B- cells, T-cells, liver, spleen, tonsils, central nervous system, enteric nervous system

The CB1 Receptor is the most common G protein receptor found in the human brain. Highest densities found in the hippocampus, cerebral cortex, cerebellum, amygdala nucleus, basal ganglia. The functions of these areas of the brain account for the effects of Hemp on short-term memory, cognition, mood and emotion, motor function, nociception. Cannabinoid receptors are virtually absent in brainstem cardiorespiratory centers meaning there's –
NO LETHAL OVERDOSE!

Neural Plasticity

Involves the sprouting and pruning of synapses; changes in dendritic spine density and changes neurotransmitter pathways, gives rise to all types of adaptive learning such as recovering after a stroke and the conscious act of learning a new skill or unconscious acquisition of new emotional response or a pathological process central sensitization for pain.

Ways by which cannabinoids modulate neural plasticity include neurogenesis and the formation of new neurons. From the Department of Health and Human Services on a patent on the use of cannabinoids as antioxidants and neuroprotectants: the author describes the benefits of using cannabinoids in neurodegenerative conditions such as Alzheimer's, Parkinson's, Huntington's, multiple sclerosis, etc.

Endocannabinoid System and Pain

The functioning of this system is the 'first line of defense' against pain. The Endocannabinoid System is heavily involved in pain signaling.

Endocannabinoids in Bone

Stimulating CB2 receptors increases bone formation, CB1 allows bone to form. Increasing bone density and mass.

Immune System

Cannabinoids modulate the immune system. Phytocannabinoids have other immune mediating effects on the body. Human breast milk has cannabinoids present. CBD Oil is given to 6 week old babies with astounding results.

Hemp and Cancer

Melanoma cancer cells actually have receptors on them that cause apoptosis when they come in contact with CBDs.

- Anti-proliferative prevents the spread and growth of new tumors.

- Angiogenesis prevents the spread of new blood vessels which is how tumors grow.

- Anti-metastatic prevents tumors from breaking apart and growing in other parts of the body

- Apoptosis causes the cancer cell to kill itself.

THC's Special Abilities

- Kills cancer cells

- Causes Apoptosis, Cell Suicide, Instant Death

- Anti-proliferative prevents spread and growth of tumors

- Lasts longer than our own cannabinoids.

Entourage Effect

First introduced in 1998. Dr. EB Russo discovered that full spectrum Hemp or whole plant medicine caused 2 to 4 times greater results than just THC alone. Another finding in that same study found full spectrum produced effects 330 percent higher than isolated compounds.

A single-molecule medication, an isolated compound that has been removed from its original state existing within a complex structure combined with other compounds is what pharmaceuticals are offering, oftentimes dissecting plants trying to find what molecule presents the most benefits and then trying to recreate it in the lab. This way they can patent it. You cannot patent Mother Nature, so they have to try and duplicate her molecules in a lab.

Hemp Is A Soil Purifier

…Unless the CBD oil that you are using is pressed from Hemp plants that were grown in soil that had poor quality. Hemp removes heavy metals and chemical waste from the soil, so if it's not pure, not only could it not make you feel better, but it could potentially make you sick, even. This is why when using Hemp products, organic is imperative.

Anxiety and Depression

You can ingest it, as an adaptogen, it finds the issues in your body and corrects them, how perfect is that?

For addressing anxiety and depression we recommend microdosing:

2 drops in the morning and 2 drops at night for 3 days and if you feel like you're not achieving the desired results, you can adjust the dose accordingly by adding 2 more drops in the morning and night, one or the other, etc. We recommend using for 3 days to establish what's called a baseline and then you can dose from there, or use topically by application on the thin skin by your wrists, temples, etc.

Safety Guidelines and Issues

I think the best part of Hemp is how safe it is. As I keep saying the beauty of it is the ability to play with the dosage. Because our bodies produce cannabinoids and we use them up due to stress in our environment, our dosage might require adjusting if you're going through an extremely stressful time, you might need more drops than other days, then you can

just back off once things calm down a little bit or as you start to adjust
better.

- **Non-toxic**
- **No lethal overdose**
- **No detrimental side effects**
- **Induces relaxation**
- **Muscle relaxant**
- **Given to babies 6 weeks old**
- **Safe for pets**
- **Research shows that intoxicated Cannabis drivers drove slower and veered, but stayed in their lane**

No side effects or should we say no 'direct effects?' They call them side
effects but these are direct effects of these inadequate medications.

Great For Children

CBD is a great alternative for Aderol for ADD and ADHD. Pharmaceuticals are not safe for children. How could they have been tested? This
would be unethical and illegal as we've stated.

There has been research that proved more speech and interaction with
autistic children using CBD.

Nutritional Aspects

Hemp has vitamins A, C, E naturally occurring, B complex, minerals like
zinc, potassium, calcium, iron magnesium, contains all 20 amino acids.
chlorophyll, alkanes, nitrogenous compounds, sugars, aldehydes, alco-
hols, ketones, flavonoids, glycosides, vitamins, and pigments. High in essential fatty acids and Omega 3's and 6's.

What's Wrong With The Medication Your Doctor Gives You?

Odds are whatever your doctor gives you for pain, is not good for your
liver, is addictive, shouldn't be taken for a prolonged period of time and

is temporary. Many of my patients have been able to get off of their pharmaceutical medications after using my CBD formulations, whether it's topical or sublingual, is not an indicating factor.

Both work well, I have had patients stop taking Ibuprofen, Tramadol, Gabapentin, avoid Cortisone injections, etc.

These are all conditions that I have helped my patients relieve:

- **lingering neuropathy**
- **shoulder pain**
- **slipped discs**
- **herniated, bulging discs**
- **sports injuries**
- **car accident injuries**
- **insomnia**
- **chronic back pain**
- **migraines**
- **anxiety**
- **cancer**
- **lipoma**
- **rheumatoid arthritis**
- **muscular dystrophy**
- **Lyme disease**
- **scoliosis**
- **fibromyalgia**
- **plantar fasciitis**
- **arthritis**
- **eczema**
- **psoriasis**
- **scarring**
- **migraines**
- **leg cramps**

- bruising
- swelling
- anxiety
- weight loss
- elbow pain
- knee pain
- extreme foot pain
- seizures
- energy levels
- wrist pain
- arthritic knuckles and hands
- neck pain
- hip pain
- broken rib pain
- after surgery pain
- restless leg syndrome
- incessant paw licking by dogs
- canine aggression and anxiety
- canine seizures
- canine arthritis
- canine cancer

There is nothing more rewarding for me than knowing that I helped someone part from the path of chronic pain and crossover onto the journey back to well-being. We were not meant to be in pain, we are not meant to suffer. We are meant to enjoy health and vitality, if these are just beyond your reach, or you've lost sight altogether, reach out, get in touch, let me be the light at the end of the tunnel and get the relief you've been waiting for! YOU DESERVE IT ...

Lab Testing

When choosing your medicine, make sure it is third-party laboratory tested. Many products on the market contain pesticides, herbicides, mold, fungi and dangerous mycotoxins. Use companies that utilize cutting-edge testing and world-class equipment to ensure quality, verified by GMP. GMP (stands for Good Manufacturing Practice) is a system for ensuring that products are consistently produced and controlled according to quality standards.

Research the lab...what are they certified to test for? Currently, at the time of this writing, no organization is certifying 'organic' hemp in the U.S.

Ask questions:

- **Is it organic?**
- **Growing conditions?**
- **Has it been tested?**
- **What has it been tested for?**
- **Potency?**
- **Pesticidal residues?**
- **Residual Solvents?**
- **Heavy Metals? CBD from China has been found to have high amounts of heavy metals.**
- **Should have ISO Accreditation (International Organization for Standardization) overseen by the regulatory body**

Nettle

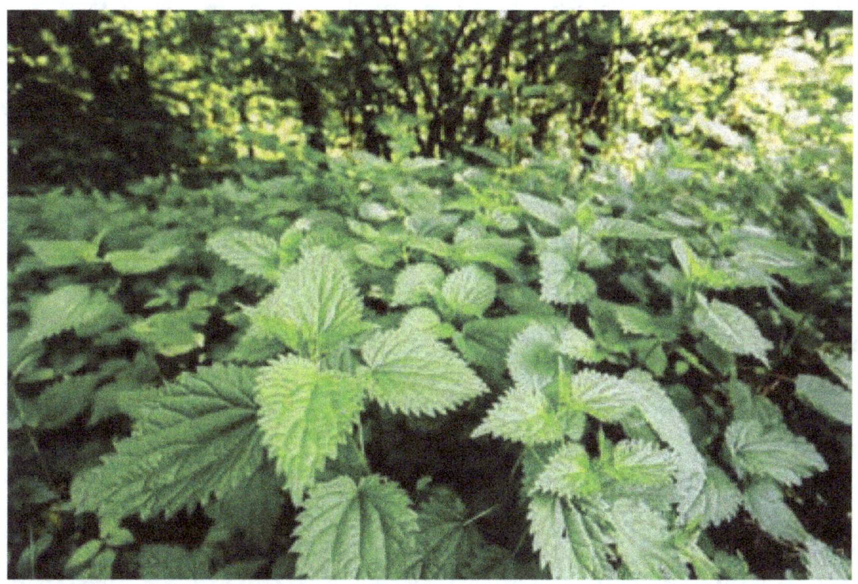

"When it sprouts fresh from the earth, it is useful cooked as food for people because it cleans and purges the stomach."

—*Hildegard Von Bingen*

Nettle - *Urtica Dioica*

In Cancer-Free Protocol

Other names: Common Nettle, Stinging Nettles

Genus: Urtica, herbaceous perennial flowering plant in the family Urticaceae

Native to colder regions of Europe, Asia, United States and Canada

Name Origin: 'Two houses' is what the latin name of the plant *dioica* means. Referring to the fact that the male and female flowers are normally carried on separate plants.

Noedl which means a needle - could be referring to the stinging mechanism in the leaves. Another possibility is that it is derived from the Latin *nere* and other similar old European verb which mean to sew.

Notes:

Galen and Dioscorides used Nettles in ancient Greece as a diuretic and laxative.

Contributory plant used in the manufacture of cloth and paper since Neolithic times.

In Medieval Europe, it was used as a diuretic and to naturally reduce joint pain.

Ancient Greeks and Romans cultivated more Nettles than any other, using it as food and medicine as well as clothing.

People used to believe pulling it out by the roots and shouting an ill person's name would eliminate a fever as well.

The German Army collected over 2,000,000 kg during World War I using it to make uniforms and the leaves for dying them.

Highly effective for enlarged prostate, a clinical study found.

Their presence in the garden indicates a nitrogen content.

Rennet substitute in homemade cheeses for vegan or vegetarian dishes.

Parts used: leaves, root, seeds

Root: Contains high amounts of sterols especially sitosterol and isolectins which stimulate white blood cell production that counteract inflammation and infection.

Seeds: Used as preventative and curative for prostate issues.

Curative Properties: amphoretic, analgesic, anti-allergic, anticancer, anticatarrhal, anticoagulant, antidiabetic, antihemorrhagic, antihistamine, antihypertensive, antiinflammatory, antimicrobial, antioxidant, antiscorbutic, antiulcer, antiviral, astringent, circulatory stimulant, diuretic, expectorant, galactagogue, hemostatic, hypotensive, nutritive, parasiticide, pectoral, restorative, rubefacients, stimulant, uterine tonic, vasodilator

Energy and flavors: cool, bland, slightly bitter

Cautions:

1. Pregnant women should not use until last weeks of pregnancy.

2. Leaves sting when lightly touched, fresh plants can cause mild to severe rash, this sting is destroyed by heating, drying or mashing. Rubbing some freshly bruised leaves of Plantain or Yellow Dock over the area is a good treatment for Nettle rash.

According to Dr. Axe: "Possible contraindications - check with your Healthcare Provider if taking these medications:

- Blood thinners, such as Warfarin, Clopidogrel and aspirin, do not use because Stinging Nettle contains large amounts of vitamin K, which can help the blood's ability to clot, but taking Stinging Nettle can decrease the effects of these drugs.

- High blood pressure medications such as ACE inhibitors, beta-blockers and calcium channel blockers are not recommended. Stinging Nettle can lower blood pressure and strengthen the effects of these drugs.

- Avoid if taking diuretics and water pills because Stinging Nettle is also a diuretic and when used together can cause dehydration.

- Lithium because of Stinging Nettle's diuretic qualities. It may reduce the body's ability to remove this drug, resulting in higher than recommended levels of lithium.

- Sedative medications (CNS depressants) such as Clonazepam, Lorazepam, Phenobarbital and Zolpidem because when large amounts of above ground parts of Stinging Nettles are taken, sleepiness and drowsiness can occur. Taking sedatives along with Stinging Nettle might cause too much drowsiness."

Conditions: allergies, anemia, arthritis, asthma, benign prostatic hyperplasia, bladder infections, bronchial problems, burns, cancer, chronic arthritic, creaky joints in old folks, cystitis, dysentery, eczema, enlarged prostate, fertility issues, fever, gout, growing pains in children, hay fever, heavy menstrual bleeding, hemorrhoids, hormonal imbalance, hyperuricemia, insect bites, menopause, menstruating difficulties, nephritis, neuralgia, painful muscles and joints, PMS, rheumatoid arthritis, sciatica, sprains, swollen joints, tendonitis, urinary complaints (chronic or acute), urinary issues, urinary stones, urinary tract infections, wounds

Biochemical constituents: chlorophyll, acetylcholine, vitamin C, vitamin A and other important vitamins, silicon, potassium, protein fiber, iron, mucilage, ammonia, carbonic acid, formic acid, serotonin, histamine

Leaves: stinging hairs: vitamin K, beta carotene, protein, potassium, calcium, flavonoids, bicarbonate of ammonia is what stings, destroyed with heat, drying or mashing

Parts of the body: bladder, lungs, reproductive system of both women and men, small intestines, urinary tract

Preparations~

Heavy Bleeding:
Sprinkling powder on wound helps to stop bleeding or
Heat Nettles for 30 minutes and squeeze them through a cloth.
Take 1 tbs. of this every hour to stop bleeding.

Asthma and Bronchial problems:
Breathing in the burning dried leaves is a home treatment for asthma and bronchial problems.

Endometriosis or Uterine Bleeding:

Infusion:
Blend equal parts:
Nettle leaf
Agrimony
Bayberry
Cinnamon
Steep in simmering water for 20 minutes.

Dose:
Take 1/2 cup full every hour tapering off as bleeding subsides.

Whole Body Toning Tincture:
Take 10 to 30 drops of tincture as a tonic.

Multivitamin Blood Purifying Tea:
Most nutritious plant in the plant kingdom.

Dose:
1 8 oz. cup of tea a day

Scalp wash:
Boil 3 to 4 oz. chopped leaves
1 cup of water and 2 cups of vinegar for a short time
Rinse scalp

Astringent Gargle:
Diluted ½ and ½ with water to fresh juice.

Rheumatic Pain:
Rub raw leaves directly on pain to increase circulation and draw
out pain.

Hair Toning Rinse for Dandruff or Alopecia:
1 tsp. leaves
1 cup hot water
Steep 10 minutes

Rinse
Stimulates hair growth when applied to the scalp

Urtication:
Ancient practice of flogging oneself with branches for swollen joints and to improve circulation.
Clears uric acid.

Recipe~

Spring Nettle Leaf Stir Fry:
Fresh young leaves should be harvested no more than 6 inches long when gathered.
Chop, add butter and pepper to taste, sauté.
Added alongside broccoli, parsley, basil, leeks or onions for a vegetable casserole with rice.
Cooked Nettle is a great source of vitamins A, C, protein and iron.

More Information: So many uses around the house and farm. Hung outside the kitchen door, keeps flies away. Can be combined with hay and fed to cattle to increase milk yield. Increases laying in hens when fed dried and powdered. Seeds can be mixed with food to increase the glossiness of dogs' and horses' coats. Its high vitamin C content ensures iron is properly absorbed by the body.

I was introduced to this plant when I was pregnant with my first daughter, Cherisse, and my amazing Midwife, Judy Luce, told me to start drinking Nettle leaf tea a month before my due date to ensure the clotting of my blood after giving birth.

High in vitamin K, Nature's hemostatic, remember I said, "Nature is Divine?" Even a plant to stop bleeding? And Nettle isn't the only one, there are others, but Nettle is my 'go-to' for vitamin K as well as a whole host of other vitamins, being the most nutritious plant in the plant kingdom.

I used to give it to my girls every day when they were little as a vitamin, a cup a day. Because of its action of drying up mucus, if my grandson starts sniffling or first signs of a cough, we have a cup of Nettle tea. We also utilized Nettle's healing properties for my husband when he was suffering from cancer, drinking it every day. Definitely one of the plants I am grateful for and attribute his phenomenal healing to.

Summary ~

After reading this book, we are clear as to the importance of reading labels, before administering anything to our children. We are aware of the seedy toy industry and how we can't just give our child a toy from anywhere, for their health's sake, it's really important to know what the materials are that the toy was made from. Which can be a little uncomfortable when people give your children toxic toys.

One idea is to give the grandparents links to the companies you like and direct them to purchase gifts from these websites. If you told them why, how could they disagree? Remember about your dollar being your voice, maybe if you stop buying poison, they will be forced to stop making it!

We know that there are herbs that cannot only stimulate lactation but increase it as well. We are now aware of the toxic carcinogenic ingredients found in our baby's bottle, sippy cups, etc. And fully grasp the comparisons of data in how our child's life literally depends on if they are breastfed or artificially fed and if we choose to use formula, we now have choices for a better formula, if we so choose.

We understand the risks involved with giving children under 2 years old cow's milk and how cow's milk is actually not necessarily as good for our children as we are led to believe, known to cause allergies and that some fruits and veggies in place of dairy and milk products in their diet might be wiser choices for our families.

Understanding the role of the immune system and how disease works, we are now equipped to boost our child's immunity instead of lowering it with pharmaceuticals. We know they will always be a last resort for the health and vitality of your child.

We understand the safety and efficacy of CBD Oil and how this choice would be much safer for our children. We understand the risks involved in injecting our children with diseases grown on animals and eggs and the way they work in our body intermingling with our DNA and how they are linking vaccines with autoimmune diseases.

The concept that what disease is in the shot isn't even the worst of your worries, how they are prepared with toxins such as formaldehyde, mercury and aluminum that can cause a myriad of symptoms in our children, is yet another factor to consider.

Don't just believe me. Ask your doctor before he injects your child. What are the ingredients in the vaccine? Is it a live virus? One child received a live polio vaccine, years ago, who lived with an elderly relative who contracted polio and died.

Ask if it's a live virus. Look at the ingredients...you need answers to these questions. It is your right. Informed consent, many doctors' offices are implementing this practice now after learning the risks and dangers involved with vaccines.

So even if the idea of vaccines was a propensity, who is going to condone mixing them with formaldehyde, mercury and aluminum? When the idea of vaccines was introduced, they didn't say, "We'll save so many lives by injecting children and babies with formaldehyde, mercury and aluminum??"

That wasn't part of the immunization method, it's the disease that's supposed to build immunity. Formaldehyde, mercury and aluminum aren't any immune boosters that I am aware of. So right there that blows the whole premise for it being ok.

We understand that there has been an unnecessary loss of life leaving our children at the mercy of Big Pharma. We can believe me when I say that I am merely trying to bring awareness to practices and protocols that I couldn't believe existed when I found out about them and my obligation as a parent to another parent as a human being to another human being for the sake of humanity is to tell you what I know, to pass on the knowledge as it has been handed down that I have utilized to protect my family and I hope this information helps you protect yours, too!

www.ingramcontent.com/pod-product-compliance
Lightning Source LLC
Chambersburg PA
CBHW060911140726
47996CB00001B/205